Illustrated Insights in Sleep
Excessive Sleepiness

Stephen M. Stahl, MD, PhD

Edited by
Christine M. Higgins, MS

Illustrations by
Nancy Muntner

NEI Press

San Diego, CA

Published by NEI Press
San Diego CA 92008
http://www.neiglobal.com

Printed in the United States of America

Typeset in Myriad Web

ISBN 1-4225-0018-7

Table of Contents

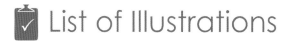 List of Illustrations

Module 1

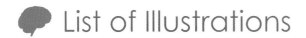 List of Illustrations

List of Illustrations

Preface to the *Illustrated Insights* Collection

Welcome to *Illustrated Insights*, a unique collection of books published by NEI Press. Books in this series describe the neurobiological basis of psychiatric disorders and their treatments by utilizing the unique didactic style that we have developed over the years, namely combining easy to read text with informative illustrations. *Illustrated Insights in Sleep* is a multi-volume collection that provides clinicians with a simple yet comprehensive resource that examines common sleep disorders. The volume presented here specifically covers those sleep disorders associated with excessive sleepiness. Other volumes in the sleep series deal with insomnia and circadian rhythm disorders.

A major theme of the *Illustrated Insights* collection is to help the reader treat patients by attaining an understanding of the circuits underlying the symptoms of the disorder being treated. This involves not only having a clear understanding of the symptoms the patient is having, but also knowing how malfunction of neurobiological circuits leads to these symptoms, and thus, how different pharmacological agents acting on these circuits can treat the problem by removing the symptom.

A Groundbreaking Learning Tool

Each book in the *Illustrated Insights* collection is divided into three modules: Diagnosis, Neurobiology, and Treatment. Each module begins with a list of objectives and a clinical question that lies at the heart of the material presented in the module. These two elements prompt the reader to preview the concepts that will be encountered and explored in the reading. Each module concludes with a summary of the main points and provides an answer to the clinical question posed at the start—elements that prompt the reader to *rehearse, review*, and *reflect*—driving home the concepts emphasized within the module.

The reader will delve into the concepts within each module by studying a series of richly illustrated, two- or four-page spreads, each spread telling a concise and complete story within the context and framework of the rest of the module. The unique design of the two- or four-page spreads will appeal to the diverse learning needs of readers.

- Rich visual elements…Visual learners will appreciate the wealth of figures, accompanied by highly descriptive and self-contained legends that enable these linked, visual bullets of information to tell a coherent story and stand alone: the visual learner will have sufficient detail and information to understand the material by simply reviewing the figures and their legends.

- Concise storylines…The more verbal or linguistic learner will appreciate the running narrative subtext that binds each two- or four-page spread and provides a more detailed and cohesive discussion of the subject matter.
- Linked information…Nonlinear learners and thinkers will appreciate bullets of information (or asides), presented in gray boxes thoughtfully juxtaposed to the related topics discussed within the main flow of the narrative.
- A problem-solving learning paradigm…Interactive learners will appreciate the Sleep Detective exercise; that is, the clinical question posed at the beginning of each module. These exercises encourage the reader to preview the module and to probe for the answers to the clinical questions in the course of reading the module. At the end of each module, an answer to the question is provided.
- Repetition and reinforcement…Concepts are introduced and previewed at the start of each module; explored in depth through a sequence of graphics and narrative storylines; and finally reviewed, rehearsed, and reinforced at the conclusion of each module. Repetition, reinforcement, and interactive elements, such as the Sleep Detective, aid the reader in learning complex concepts.

Novices to the field may choose to approach this text by going through each module from beginning to end, by first previewing the key concepts, reflecting on the Sleep Detective, and then by launching into the heart of the module, focusing only on the color graphics and their corresponding legends. Virtually everything that is covered in the text is also covered in the graphics. After completing this initial visual foray into the heart of the subject, the reader may now go back to the beginning of the module and read the narrative storylines that connect figure to figure, concept to concept, and attempt to resolve, while studying the module, the questions posed in the Sleep Detective. At the conclusion of the module, the reader can actively rehearse the concepts by reviewing each summary point while scanning the graphics one more time, and then finish by reading and contemplating the answer to the Sleep Detective. Thus, the reader is compelled to reinforce (once again!) what was learned.

Good luck on your exciting and illustrated venture into neurobiology, psychopharmacology, and psychiatry.

Stephen M. Stahl

Stephen M. Stahl, M.D., Ph.D.

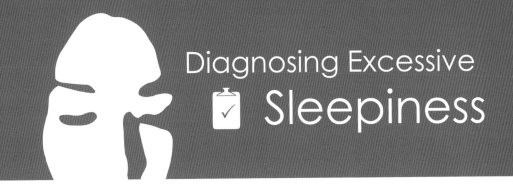

Diagnosing Excessive Sleepiness

OBJECTIVES

- List the sleep disorders that have symptoms of excessive sleepiness

- Name other medical conditions that may present symptoms of excessive sleepiness

- Explain the impact of untreated sleepiness on society and discuss when sleepiness symptoms should be pharmacologically treated in patients

- Recognize the key diagnostic features of narcolepsy, obstructive sleep apnea, and primary hypersomnia

- Describe the characteristics and potential causes of the "deficit syndrome"

CLINICAL APPLICATIONS

Cosmetic Psychopharmacology?
Excessive sleepiness is a real problem that not only affects the health and safety of the individual, but also affects all of society.

⚲ Sleep Detective
Robert is a slightly overweight 42-year-old man whose wife constantly complains of his loud snoring. Robert is being sued for reckless driving after crashing his car into his neighbor's house. He says he fell asleep at the wheel. As an expert witness for Robert, give your medical opinion of what most likely led to his accident.

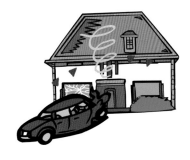

Sleepiness and Sleep Disorders

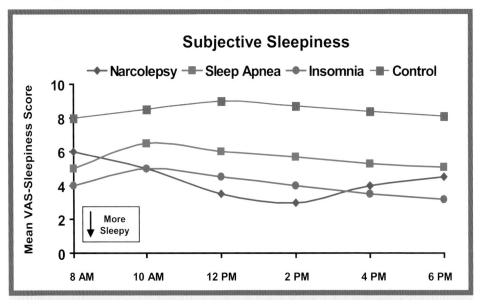

Figure 1.1 Excessive sleepiness is the primary symptom of patients diagnosed with common sleep disorders. This graph shows that the subjective level of sleepiness is significantly greater in patients with narcolepsy, insomnia, or sleep apnea compared with a control group of normal sleepers (data from Schneider et al. 2004). Increased sleepiness translates into poor work performance, a higher risk for accidents, and a reduced quality of life.

Sleep is a primary physiological need for all animals. When this need is not met, or when the neurobiological circuits underlying sleep and wakefulness are not functioning properly, excessive sleepiness can occur. The purpose of this handbook is to address the growing need for all clinicians to be aware of the symptoms, diagnostic features, and treatments of sleep disorders characterized by excessive sleepiness. In this first module, we will discuss the impact of sleepiness on patients and society, as well as how to assess excessive sleepiness and recognize common sleep disorders in patients with these symptoms.

Epidemiological data suggest approximately five percent of the general population experience excessive sleepiness. Excessive sleepiness is clinically defined as sleepiness that occurs at a time when the individual would usually be awake and alert. The term sleepiness is commonly used to describe mental fatigue, physical tiredness, or attention difficulties; however, these symptoms should not be confused with each other. Sleepiness is the propensity to fall asleep, while fatigue is a general lack of energy that is not relieved by increased sleep. Fatigue occurs more frequently in psychiatric disorders while sleepiness is indicative of sleep disorders, although there is a large degree of overlap.

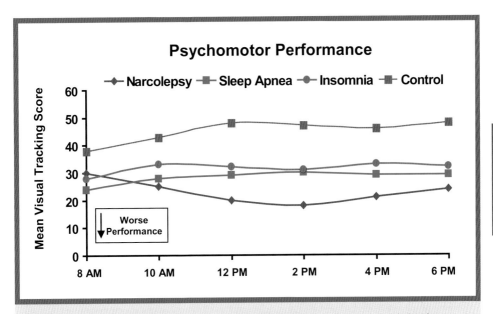

Figure 1.2 Poor performance in sleep disorders correlates with higher levels of sleepiness. Patients with narcolepsy, insomnia, or sleep apnea perform worse on a visual tracking task than a control group of normal sleepers (data from Schneider et al. 2004). Treating excessive sleepiness in sleep disorders often alleviates performance deficits.

Sleep disorders can be divided into four main categories: primary sleep disorders, those related to a mental disorder, those due to a general medical condition, and substance-induced sleep disorders (*Diagnostic and Statistical Manual of Mental Disorders, Fourth Edition*). A common clinical myth is that primary sleep disorders are usually due to lifestyle choices and can generally be treated without drugs. Another common myth promotes the viewpoint that secondary sleep disorders should only be treated by eliminating the underlying primary condition. In reality, the symptom of sleepiness often persists and may require pharmacologic treatment since lifestyle interventions and treatment of the underlying condition often fail to remove this symptom. ~

Effects of Sleepiness

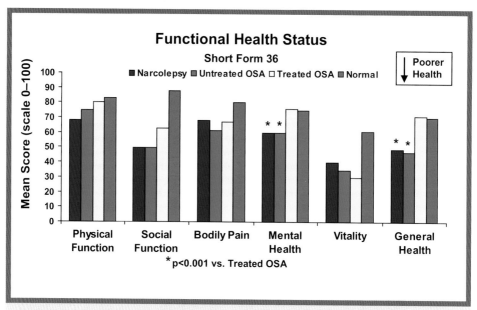

Figure 1.3 The Short Form 36 is a self-administered questionnaire that is widely used to measure subjective health status. Patients with narcolepsy (receiving stimulant treatment) or untreated obstructive sleep apnea (OSA) reported experiencing a worse overall health status than OSA patients treated with continuous positive airway pressure (CPAP) or compared with mean scores for the general healthy population (Teixeira et al. 2004).

The issue of cosmetic treatment of sleep problems has been pervasive within the medical community. Concerns about treating patients who do not have a true medical condition are justified. The treatment for sleepiness due to sleep deprivation from partying or overwork is sleep, not a drug. Individuals who have sleepiness due to running up their sleep debt in this manner should not be treated pharmacologically since this will only drive them deeper into sleep debt and reinforce poor sleep habits.

On the other hand, untreated sleepiness due to sleep disorders increases the morbidity and mortality risk for the patients. For example, patients with obstructive sleep apnea (OSA; also referred to as obstructive sleep apnea-hypopnea syndrome), are at increased risk for stroke, cardiovascular disease, hypertension, and the metabolic syndrome. The rate of mortality is significantly higher among these patients, which can be attributed to both clinical comorbidity and fatal accidents. A large body of evidence shows that identification and treatment of OSA lowers

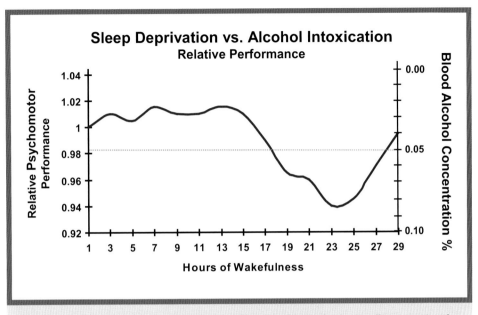

Figure 1.4 Impairment under the influence of alcohol is well recognized; however, the degree of impairment due to sleepiness is usually underappreciated. In this study, the level of performance on a visual tracking task during prolonged wakefulness was compared with performance under the influence of alcohol in the same group of participants. These data demonstrate that 24 hours of sleep deprivation (i.e., pulling an "all-nighter") can impair an individual's level of functioning to the same degree as being moderately intoxicated (Dawson et al. 1997).

the associated risks (Krieger et al. 1997; Sassani et al. 2004). Narcolepsy and other sleep disorders with excessive daytime sleepiness are similarly associated with an increased susceptibility to accidents and a poorer overall health status (Teixeira et al. 2004).

The impact of excessive sleepiness is not limited to the afflicted individual—automobile accidents, work and industrial accidents, and related healthcare costs affect society as a whole. Estimates of the total economic cost of excessive sleepiness fall between $20 billion and $100 billion annually. People with untreated OSA, narcolepsy, or other disorders with excessive sleepiness are more likely to be involved in an automobile- or work-related accident than the general public and to incur higher healthcare-related costs. It is important for clinicians to recognize the risks of untreated sleepiness and the benefits of available treatment options in order to judge which patients should receive treatment. ~

Clinical Measures of Sleepiness

The Epworth Sleepiness Scale

How likely are you to doze off or fall asleep in the following situations, in contrast to just feeling tired? This refers to your usual way of life in recent times. Even if you have not done some of these things recently, try to work out how they would have affected you. Use the following scale to choose the most appropriate number for each situation:

0= Would never doze
1= Slight chance of dozing

2= Moderate chance of dozing
3= High chance of dozing

Situation	Chance of Dozing
Sitting and reading	_____
Watching TV	_____
Sitting, inactive, in a public place (e.g., a theater or a meeting)	_____
As a passenger in a car for an hour without a break	_____
Lying down to rest in the afternoon when circumstances permit	_____
Sitting and talking to someone	_____
Sitting quietly after a lunch without alcohol	_____
In a car, while stopped for a few minutes in traffic	_____

Figure 1.5 The Epworth Sleepiness Scale is a self-rating subjective measure of sleepiness. It is useful as a point-of-care tool for rapidly assessing the severity of sleepiness in a patient. This scale is also often used in clinical studies for comparison and outcomes measurements.

While noting the number of times a patient yawns during a consultation may be a crude way to measure their sleepiness, more sophisticated methods are just as simple and much more reliable. When a patient indicates symptoms of excessive sleepiness, it is important to get a sleep history from the patient and to ask questions related to mood and to other medical conditions. In many cases, having the patient keep a sleep diary for a week can be useful in assessing the contribution of poor sleep hygiene or medication use to a person's sleep problems. Examples of a sleep health questionnaire and a patient sleep diary can be found in the back.

The Epworth Sleepiness Scale, the Visual Analog Scale for Sleepiness, the Karolinska Sleepiness Scale, and the Stanford Sleepiness Scale are examples of self-rating measures of sleepiness. These are popular scales because they can be administered outside of sleep labs, and they tend to correlate well with more objective measures of sleepiness. These tools are not diagnostic alone but can be used to indicate if further sleep evaluation is necessary.

If a primary sleep disorder such as narcolepsy, restless legs syndrome, or sleep apnea is suspected, the patient should be referred to a sleep clinic for confirmation

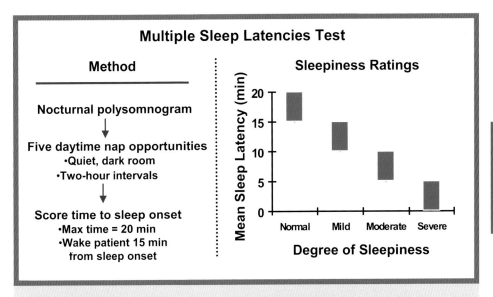

Figure 1.6 The Multiple Sleep Latencies Test (MSLT) is the most commonly used method for diagnosing sleep disorders. The test requires polysomnography equipment and must be performed by trained physicians in an accredited sleep lab. The degree of sleepiness is measured as the latency to the onset of any stage of sleep, with a mean latency of less than 10 minutes usually indicating excessive sleepiness related to a sleep disorder.

with polysomnogram. For diagnosing sleep disorders of excessive sleepiness, the Multiple Sleep Latencies Test (MSLT) is the gold standard. After a normal night of sleep in the lab (up to eight hours), patients are given five opportunities to nap in a quiet, dark room every two hours throughout the day while their latency to fall asleep is recorded by electroencephalography (EEG). Well-rested individuals normally fall asleep in 15 to 20 minutes under these conditions. Shorter sleep latencies indicate excessive sleepiness, and a mean latency of less than 10 minutes is common in many sleep disorders. The pervasiveness of chronic sleepiness in society today can be gauged with the "poor man's" MSLT— a simple observation of how long it takes heads to drop forward during a long, boring lecture or while taxiing before take-off in an airplane. ~

Diagnosing Obstructive Sleep Apnea

Diagnostic Features

- Sleep disruption leading to excessive sleepiness
  - MSLT latency <10 min.
- Episodes of breathing cessation or slowing during sleep
  - Measured as RDI ≥5 per hour
- Loud snoring
- Unrefreshing sleep or naps
- Severe dry mouth and morning headaches after waking

Figure 1.7 Diagnostic features common in obstructive sleep apnea (OSA) are listed here. The respiratory disturbance index (RDI) measures the number of apneic events per hour and is considered the most important criterion for a diagnosis. Patients usually have accompanying sleepiness ranging from mild to severe due to disrupted sleep.

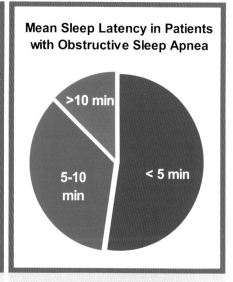

Mean Sleep Latency in Patients with Obstructive Sleep Apnea

>10 min

5-10 min

< 5 min

Figure 1.8 MSLT scores in patients with a diagnosis of OSA are moderate to severe (i.e., less than 10 minutes) in 82% of patients. Patients with mild sleepiness may still have other problems associated with their apnea, such as cognitive impairment.

Sleep apnea is becoming a well-known medical condition among the public. This is in part due to increased acknowledgment of the disorder in the medical community, and in part due to an increased prevalence as the population ages and waistlines expand. OSA is a sleep disorder in which the upper airway is partially or fully obstructed during sleep, causing brief apnea events lasting 10–30 seconds on average. OSA is diagnosed when excessive sleepiness occurs in combination with at least five apnea events per hour during sleep, defined by the respiratory disturbance index (RDI). The apnea events cause significant sleep disruption leading to unrefreshing sleep and residual daytime sleepiness. Other daytime symptoms include poor concentration, decreased attention, depressed mood, and fatigue. Some of these daytime symptoms may be attributed to executive dysfunction in OSA patients, due to impairment of the prefrontal cortex.

Research on the risk factors and health outcomes of OSA has continuously run into the "chicken or the egg" problem. Obesity is the strongest risk factor for OSA, estimated to be present in 60–90% of patients diagnosed with the disorder

Risk Factors	Executive Dysfunction in OSA
• Overweight • Male • Over 40 years old • History of snoring • Hypertension • Hypothyroidism	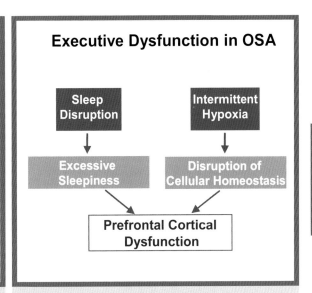

Figure 1.9 OSA is most commonly diagnosed in overweight men and the elderly. In children, undiagnosed OSA may lead to many of the same behavioral and cognitive problems as attention deficit hyperactivity disorder (ADHD).

Figure 1.10 Executive functions, such as working memory and complex problem solving, are particularly vulnerable to sleep disturbances. Since patients with OSA also experience brief episodes of hypoxia as well as sleep disruptions throughout the night, they are especially likely to experience executive dysfunction.

(Bassari and Guillement, 2000), but it is unclear if obesity is causal or incidental to OSA. Hypertension is found in over 40% of patients with OSA (Baguet et al. 2005); however, there is debate about whether OSA leads to hypertension, or vice versa. Many of the factors associated with OSA (hypertension, asthma, heart disease, diabetes) are also associated with obesity, and the independent association of these factors with OSA is still being determined. Several studies have shown that weight loss significantly reduces the number of apnea events, and in many cases, eliminates the need for alternative treatment (Sanders, 2000).

Virtually all patients with OSA snore, and most have a history of snoring for many years. Snoring that gets progressively louder or more frequent often precedes the onset of daytime sleepiness in patients who develop OSA. In children, loud snoring and poor performance at school may indicate childhood sleep apnea, which affects between one and three percent of school-age children and is behaviorally similar to attention deficit hyperactivity disorder. ∼

Diagnosing Hypersomnia

Diagnostic Features of Narcolepsy

- Severe daytime sleepiness
  - Frequent lapses into unintentional sleep
  - Two or more SOREMP during MSLT; latency <10 min.
- Episodes of cataplexy
  - Present in over 2/3 of narcoleptic patients
- Sleep paralysis
- Hypnagogic and hypnopompic hallucinations
  - Common during daytime sleep attacks

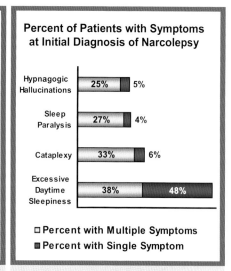

Percent of Patients with Symptoms at Initial Diagnosis of Narcolepsy

	Percent with Multiple Symptoms	Percent with Single Symptom
Hypnagogic Hallucinations	25%	5%
Sleep Paralysis	27%	4%
Cataplexy	33%	6%
Excessive Daytime Sleepiness	38%	48%

Figure 1.11 Cataplexy is considered the defining feature of narcolepsy and alone is sufficient for a diagnosis. Narcolepsy frequently occurs without cataplexy though, so an MSLT is always recommended as a diagnostic measure. Patients with narcolepsy will often fall directly into REM sleep rather than progressing through other sleep stages. Two of these sleep-onset REM periods (SOREMPs) are required for a diagnosis of narcolepsy.

Figure 1.12 Excessive daytime sleepiness (EDS) is the most common reason narcoleptic patients seek medical help and are diagnosed. According to one retrospective study, at the time of initial diagnosis, 79% of all narcoleptic patients experienced EDS, and it was the only symptom in 48% of patients (Morrish et al. 2004).

Narcolepsy is a disorder of inappropriate sleep/wake transitions, while hypersomnia denotes an underlying problem with arousal. The typical clinical features of narcolepsy include excessive sleepiness and cataplexy, but sleep paralysis and hypnagogic or hypnopompic hallucinations are also frequent, and the symptoms can occur in any combination. Sleep paralysis is a frightening state in which the patient remains conscious but is completely unable to move upon falling asleep or waking. Sleep paralysis is often accompanied by visual hallucinations which are vivid, often scary, dream-like images that occur either when falling asleep (hypnagogic) or when awakening (hypnopompic). In many patients, new symptoms will develop over time. One study found that while only nine percent of patients had all four clinical features upon initial diagnosis, over half of long-term narcoleptics had the tetrad of features (Morrish et al. 2004).

Narcolepsy is due to a loss of function of the peptide neurotransmitter called hypocretin (also known as orexin). An autoimmune process in genetically vulnerable individuals, particularly those with HLA (human leukocyte antigen)

Primary Hypersomnia

Differential Diagnosis

- Substance-induced
  - Drug of abuse
  - Medication use
  - Exposure to a toxin
- Psychiatric disorder
  - Major depressive disorder
  - Depressed phase of bipolar disorder
- Sleep deprivation
  - Symptoms reversed with increased sleep
- Posttraumatic hypersomnia
  - Head trauma
  - CNS injury
- Delay- or advance-phase sleep syndrome
  - Circadian rhythm is shifted

Diagnostic Measures in Narcolepsy and Hypersomnia

	ESS	MSLT Lat. (min)	MSLT # SO-REMP	CSF Hypo-cretin pg/ml
Narcolepsy with Cataplexy	18	3.38	3.5	96.5
Narcolepsy without Cataplexy	19	2.75	2.5	277.3
Primary Hyper-somnia	17	6	0	226.8
Hyper-somnia in Psychiatric Disorders	18	7.83	0	278

(data from Bassetti et al 2003)

Figure 1.13 Differential diagnosis in patients with hypersomnia disorders can be very difficult, but is important in choosing the best treatment. The diagnosis of primary hypersomnia is reserved for those patients in whom no other factor can be considered causal to the symptom of sleepiness.

DQB1*0602 and DQA1*0102 (Mignot et al. 1994), is suspected of causing degeneration of the hypothalamic neurons that produce hypocretin. In a few cases, mutations or polymorphisms of the prehypocretin gene have been found in individuals with narcolepsy (Gencik et al. 2001). It is interesting to note that narcolepsy without cataplexy (roughly 30% of narcoleptics) is not associated with reduced hypocretin CSF levels. Narcoleptic patients with cataplexy, but without the DQB1*0602 allele (around 6%–15%), also tend to have normal levels of hypocretin, suggesting multiple pathologies of this disorder (Krahn et al. 2002). It may be that other aspects of hypocretin signaling (such as receptor insensitivity) play a role in cases of narcolepsy without clear hypocretin deficiencies.

Primary hypersomnia is presumed to be due to a biological malfunction in the brain's arousal circuits, but a clear basis for the condition is unknown. A diagnosis of primary hypersomnia is only given to patients with moderate to severe sleepiness that has no other known cause. Hypersomnia is frequently seen in psychiatric disorders, and in these cases, treatment for both the primary disorder and excessive sleepiness may be necessary. ~

The "Deficit Syndrome"

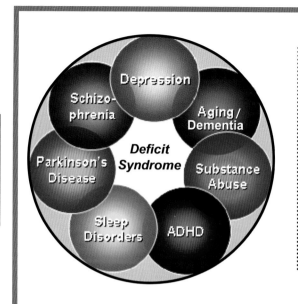

Deficit Symptoms

• Fatigue

• Lack of motivation

• Emotional blunting

• Loss of vitality

• Diminished goal-directedness

• Memory problems

Figure 1.14 The "deficit syndrome" is a term applied to a general state of executive dysfunction, often associated with a subjective sense of fatigue and sometimes referred to as chronic fatigue syndrome. Executive function is especially challenged in individuals with excessive sleepiness, whether it is a symptom of a sleep disorder, mood disorder, or other conditions. In such cases, patients with sleep disorders may need treatment with an agent that targets executive function in order to return to a normal level of functioning.

Symptoms of fatigue, anhedonia, and memory problems associated with sleepiness may indicate a condition clinically referred to as the "deficit syndrome." This syndrome is a collection of enduring symptoms related to impaired prefrontal cortical function, especially in the dorsolateral prefrontal cortex (DLPFC). Symptoms of the "deficit syndrome" often accompany psychiatric and sleep disorders. It is presumed that symptoms result from disrupted monoaminergic and/or histaminergic neurotransmission, since drugs that alter the activity of these neurotransmitters are effective in treating many of these symptoms. It is not surprising that excessive sleepiness is commonly associated with symptoms of the "deficit syndrome" since the prefrontal cortex is particularly sensitive to sleep disruption (Verstraeten and Cluydts, 2004).

Patients with excessive sleepiness should be assessed for other symptoms of the "deficit syndrome." In sleep disorders, improved sleep quality or sleep duration through treatment will usually alleviate these symptoms. If symptoms do persist after treatment, alternative or augmenting pharmacological treatment options that specifically target these residual symptoms should be considered in order to

Overlap of Symptoms in Sleep and Psychiatric Disorders

| | Disorder | | | | |
Symptom	Major Depressive Disorder	Attention Deficit Hyperactivity Disorder	Narcolepsy	Obstructive Sleep Apnea	Shift-Work Sleep Disorder
Mood	+++	-	-	+	-
Sleepiness	+	+	+++	+++	+++
Fatigue	++	+	++	++	++
Concentration	++	+++	++	++	++

+++ Most Common   ++ Common   + Average   - None

Figure 1.15 Many of the symptoms seen in sleep disorders are common in psychiatric disorders and vice versa. This chart compares the frequency of different symptoms among common sleep and psychiatric disorders, which is useful in making a differential diagnosis. The degree of symptom overlap among many disorders emphasizes the need to be able to recognize and treat a patient's individual symptoms, rather than use a single treatment strategy for all symptoms of a disorder.

achieve the best outcome for the patient. Treatments for excessive sleepiness and the deficit syndrome are discussed in the final module.

Several occurrences of sleep disorders presenting as other psychiatric conditions have been highlighted in case reports, which emphasize the need for a broader understanding of the symptoms of sleep disorders within the medical profession. There are many accounts of children diagnosed with ADHD who were later discovered to actually have OSA. It is currently estimated that as many as 25% of children with ADHD have an underlying sleep problem (Chervin et al. 2002). Sleepiness due to sleep disorders has been linked to impaired concentration and inattention in both adults and children (Chervin et al. 2002; Sangal and Sangal, 2004). In other cases, narcolepsy with hypnagogic hallucinations has been mislabeled as schizophrenia (Kishi et al. 2004). It is helpful to note that in narcolepsy hallucinations are usually visual and accompany sleep attacks, while in schizophrenia, auditory hallucinations when fully awake are more likely. In patients where a schizophrenia diagnosis is questionable, an MSLT may be warranted. These examples point out the importance of asking *all* patients about their sleep history and the degree to which they experience daytime sleepiness. ~

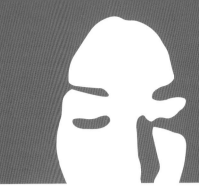

SUMMARY POINTS

- Excessive sleepiness is the primary symptom of many sleep disorders, but is also present in several other medical and psychiatric disorders

- Diagnosing the cause of excessive sleepiness is critical to a patient's long-term health and may benefit the safety of society as a whole

- There are both self-rating and objective clinical measures of sleepiness; the MSLT is the most widely used test for diagnosing sleep disorders

- Moderate to severe sleepiness can occur in many sleep disorders; a differential diagnosis is based on associated symptoms and the patient's medical and family history, in addition to their MSLT results

- The "deficit syndrome" is a final functional outcome in a wide variety of medical, mental, and sleep disorders, characterized by executive dysfunction and fatigue; excessive sleepiness is often accompanied by the other symptoms of the "deficit syndrome"

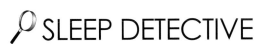
$\mathcal{P}$ SLEEP DETECTIVE

Robert is a slightly overweight 42-year-old man whose wife constantly complains of his loud snoring. Robert is being sued for reckless driving after crashing his car into his neighbor's house. He says he fell asleep at the wheel. As an expert witness for Robert, give your medical opinion of what most likely led to his accident.

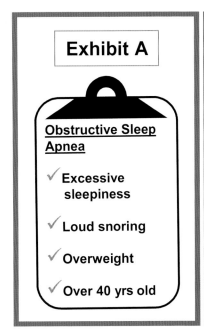

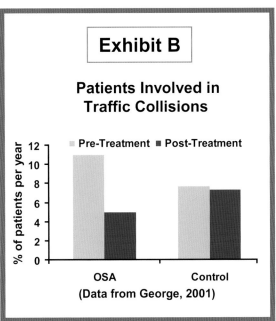

Robert's symptoms of loud snoring and falling asleep at the wheel, along with his age and weight characteristics, are highly suggestive of OSA (Exhibit A). It is estimated that three percent of drivers on the road have untreated OSA. Most people never realize they have it until something like a car crash forces them to seek medical attention. The probable reason for Robert's accident is excessive daytime sleepiness associated with undiagnosed OSA.

The good news is that with treatment, Robert's level of functioning, including his driving performance, is likely to return to normal (Exhibit B). Robert will be referred to a sleep lab for an MSLT to confirm a diagnosis of OSA. With proper treatment, his excessive sleepiness should be significantly diminished, and future accidents can be avoided.

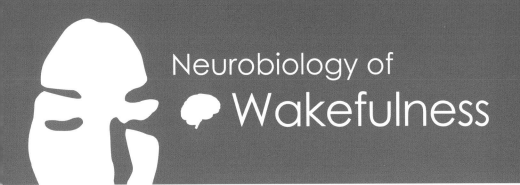

Neurobiology of Wakefulness

OBJECTIVES

- List the main neuronal circuits and the neurotransmitters that regulate wakefulness in the brain

- Discuss the role of monoamines and histamine in producing different levels of arousal and how they affect behavior

- Describe the role of hypocretin deficiency in causing excessive sleepiness and cataplexy in narcolepsy

- Explain how dopamine release varies with relative levels of arousal

- State the neurobiological region that controls executive function, and discuss why executive dysfunction often occurs with sleepiness

CLINICAL APPLICATIONS

Better Care through Better Understanding
A good understanding of the neurobiology underlying symptoms of excessive sleepiness is essential for providing patients with the best quality care.

○ Sleep Detective

George suffers from primary hyper-somnia and requires medication to treat his excessive sleepiness. His managed care provider refuses to cover the medication under the assumption that George's sleepiness does not have a biological cause. Explain to George's provider how symptoms of excessive sleepiness can arise from malfunctioning circuits in the brain.

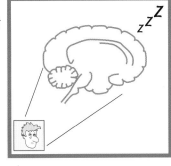

Wakefulness and Arousal

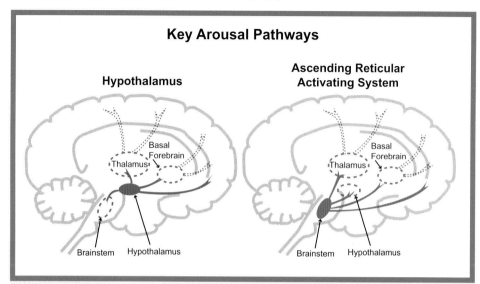

Figure 2.1 Wakefulness is a state of cortical arousal maintained by the coordination of two main arousal centers: the hypothalamus and the ascending reticular activating system (ARAS). The hypothalamus integrates information about metabolic state, memory, mood, homeostatic drives, and the environment and sends projections to the basal forebrain, brainstem, and cortex to regulate arousal. The ARAS is a heterogeneous collection of brainstem nuclei that receives somatic and visceral inputs and in turn sends excitatory and modulatory projections to subcortical and cortical structures to drive and modulate arousal.

The goal of this module is to illustrate how the brain generates wakefulness and arousal, as a foundation for understanding how pharmacological agents work on arousal circuits to treat symptoms of excessive sleepiness. Wakefulness is a state of behavioral arousal that must be actively maintained through cortical activation. Excessive sleepiness occurs when the arousal circuits are not fully functional, either because of sleep deprivation or a neurobiological cause.

Two key neural centers, the hypothalamus and the brainstem ascending reticular activating system (ARAS), drive cortical activation. A useful model for understanding the role of these centers in arousal is to view the hypothalamus as the commander, switching between states of sleep and wakefulness, while the brainstem is the manager, directing the brain through various activation stages during sleep or wakefulness. In the hypothalamus, specific populations of neurons are tonically active during wakefulness, primarily in the tuberomammillary nucleus (TMN) and the lateral hypothalamus (LH). The TMN is known as the wake-promoter, and it is essential for a state of wakefulness. When homeostatic and circadian sensors determine it is time to sleep, inhibitory projections from another hypothalamic

Neurobiology of Wakefulness

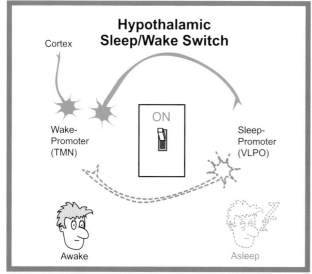

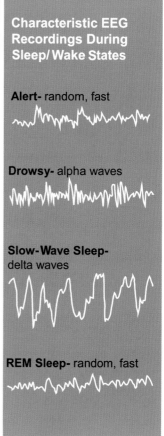

Figure 2.2 The hypothalamus is home to the sleep/wake switch. A continuous feedback loop oscillates between sleep and wake states. The tuberomammillary nucleus (TMN) is the wake-promoter, actively promoting cortical excitation while simultaneously inhibiting the sleep-promoter, the ventrolateral preoptic nucleus (VLPO). When it is time to sleep, the VLPO takes over, inhibiting the TMN to suppress wakefulness.

nucleus, the ventrolateral preoptic nucleus (VLPO, a.k.a. the sleep-promoter), shut down the TMN and LH and dim other arousal circuits.

The ARAS originates in the brainstem and consists of dorsal and ventral projections that modulate cortical activity during states of sleep or wake. The dorsal ARAS pathway goes through a thalamic relay to activate the cortex, while the ventral pathway projects to the hypothalamus and the basal forebrain, as well as directly to the frontal cortex. Most cells that comprise the ARAS receive sensory and visceral input, as well as hypothalamic and cortical feedback. Thus, the ARAS is in the position to regulate behavioral arousal based on the overall environmental and physiological picture. During sleep, the majority of brainstem neurons are inhibited by the sleep-promoter; however, there are subpopulations of cells that become active during sleep-stage transitions or during rapid eye movement (REM) sleep. This latter population drives cholinergic cells in the basal forebrain to excite the cortex, giving rise to the asynchronous neural activity that characterizes REM sleep. ~

Processes Influencing Wakefulness

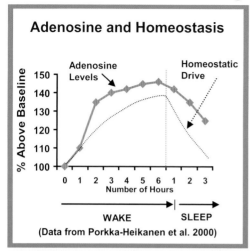

Adenosine and Homeostasis

(Data from Porkka-Heikanen et al. 2000)

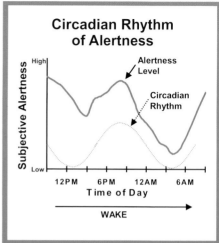

Circadian Rhythm of Alertness

Figure 2.3 There are two main processes controlling sleep/wake cycles. During wakefulness, the homeostatic drive for sleep gradually increases as the body becomes more fatigued and decreases as the body rests during sleep. Similarly, the homeostatic factor, adenosine, accumulates in the basal forebrain during prolonged wakefulness and decreases during recovery sleep in cats.

Figure 2.4 The other major process controlling the sleep/wake cycle is the endogenous circadian rhythm. Circadian influences on arousal can be seen in the average subjective alertness level of humans across a 24-hour period of wakefulness.

While many factors can influence arousal, such as hunger and activity, there are two overriding processes to consider. The homeostatic drive for sleep rises during waking periods and is relieved during sleep. In other words, a person builds up a sleep debt when awake and pays it off during sleep. It is this homeostatic drive that leads to feelings of excessive sleepiness during a state of sleep deprivation. If sleep is disrupted, such as in patients with sleep apnea, the homeostatic drive is not fully relieved and contributes to increased sleepiness the following day. This type of sleep debt may not be readily repaid through more sleep since the sleep itself is abnormal and non-restorative.

The energy metabolite, adenosine, has been hypothesized as a homeostatic regulator of sleep (Basheer et al. 2004). Prolonged wakefulness results in an accumulation of extracellular adenosine, due to the breakdown of adenosine triphosphate (ATP) during neural activity. Adenosine reduces arousal by inhibiting cholinergic projection cells in the basal forebrain and promotes sleep by indirectly activating neurons in the VLPO (the sleep-promoter). During sleep, adenosine levels decline, supporting the idea that one function of sleep is to replenish energy resources.

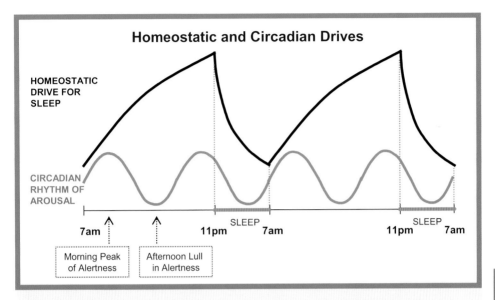

Figure 2.5 In reality, one's alertness is the sum of both homeostatic and circadian drives, determined by the time of day and one's recent sleep history. Illustrated here is the homeostatic process superimposed upon the endogenous circadian rhythm of arousal. Due to this physiological interaction, individuals are likely to feel a greater level of arousal during the morning and less arousal in the early afternoon. At night, the homeostatic drive peaks just as the circadian arousal is cycling to its lowest point, allowing one to sleep.

Circadian rhythms affect nearly all physiological systems, including body temperature, hormone release, cell proliferation, and sleep/wake cycles. Circadian influences prepare the brain to be alert during the day by augmenting activity of arousal circuits, and to rest during the night by dampening arousal circuits. This influence can easily be demonstrated during sleep deprivation; even after missing an entire night of sleep, people tend to get a "second wind" in the early morning, as the internal clock prepares the brain for daily activity. Variations in the natural circadian rhythm of individuals account for why some people are "morning-types" while others may be "night owls."

The interaction of circadian and homeostatic processes predicts how sleepy or alert a person feels throughout the day. In the morning, the circadian influence on arousal is high and the drive for sleep is low so people tend to feel very alert. The afternoon lull in alertness that most people experience is due to an increasing drive for sleep at a time when the circadian influence on arousal is low. Excessive sleepiness can occur when a person's circadian rhythm is out of sync with the sleep/wake schedule they follow, such as in shift-work sleep disorder. People with this sleep disorder have a hard time paying off their sleep debt since they are trying to sleep when circadian arousal levels are high. ∼

Arousal and Behavior

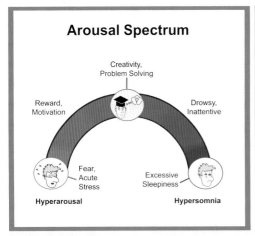

Arousal Spectrum

Creativity,
Problem Solving

Reward,
Motivation

Drowsy,
Inattentive

Fear,
Acute
Stress

Excessive
Sleepiness

Hyperarousal

Hypersomnia

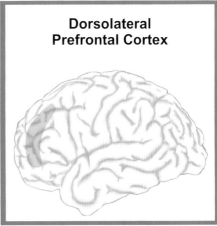

Dorsolateral Prefrontal Cortex

Figure 2.6 During wakefulness, people experience a spectrum of arousal levels ranging from hypersomnia to hyperarousal. Behavior varies along the arousal spectrum: hypersomnia is characterized by symptoms of excessive sleepiness, while hyperarousal is generally associated with fear- and stress-related behaviors, such as external vigilance and autonomic nervous system activation.

Figure 2.7 The dorsolateral prefrontal cortex (DLPFC) is a region of the brain that controls many higher-order cognitive functions that are most relevant to conscious awareness, termed executive functions. Optimal tuning of neurotransmission in cortical circuits is required for proper executive functioning.

Wakefulness in humans can be described as a state of conscious awareness that is lost during sleep. Throughout both sleep and wake states, a person experiences varying levels of arousal ranging from deep slow wave sleep to hypervigilance. The degree of arousal during wakefulness depends upon a complex orchestration of external (sensory input) and internal (thoughts, feelings) stimuli, as well as circadian and homeostatic influences.

Neurochemical evidence supports the existence of parallel pathways that activate the brain to give rise to the varying levels of arousal during wakefulness. The brainstem ARAS cholinergic, noradrenergic, and serotonergic projections stimulate cortical and subcortical regions including the thalamus, nucleus accumbens (NA), and the entire cortical mantle. In addition, descending projections from the reticular activating system activate the autonomic nervous system. The histaminergic pathway, arising from the posterior hypothalamus, excites basal forebrain cholinergic projections and can facilitate the release of monoamines within the cortex without affecting subcortical monoamine levels. Dopamine projections to

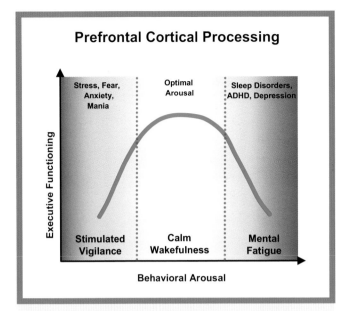

Prefrontal Cortical Processing

Stress, Fear, Anxiety, Mania

Optimal Arousal

Sleep Disorders, ADHD, Depression

Executive Functioning

Stimulated Vigilance

Calm Wakefulness

Mental Fatigue

Behavioral Arousal

Executive Functions

- Problem-solving
- Behavior modulation
- Planning and internal ordering
- Self-monitoring/ self-reflection

Executive Dysfunctions

- Disinhibited behavior
- Impaired verbal fluency
- Serial learning deficits
- Problems focusing attention
- Concentration difficulties

Figure 2.8 The DLPFC is particularly sensitive to arousal levels, and neural processing is impaired at either extreme of the arousal spectrum. Patients may experience symptoms of executive dysfunction accompanying excessive sleepiness, as in many sleep and psychiatric disorders, or when hyperstimulated, as during states of mania or extreme stress.

the NA, striatum, and prefrontal cortex (PFC) provide a third pathway that influences arousal. These neurobiological circuits work in concert to determine a person's overall level of behavioral arousal.

Many arousal-related behaviors, such as attention and locomotor activity, tend to correlate with arousal levels. However, the dorsolateral prefrontal cortex (DLPFC) is particularly sensitive to arousal levels; as a result, behaviors that are regulated by the DLPFC, i.e., executive functions such as self-reflection, planning, and decision-making, are disrupted at either end of the arousal spectrum. These behavioral differences across the arousal spectrum are likely related to the level of monoamines in cortical and subcortical areas. For DLPFC-mediated behaviors, cortical circuits must be optimally tuned to the desired neural activity. During hyperarousal, monoamines flood the brain, elevating subcortical-mediated behaviors such as motor activity, motivational state, and autonomic activation, but disrupting executive function. Conversely, during fatigue and excessive sleepiness, as in the "deficit syndrome," monoamine and histamine levels are in short supply resulting in reduced physical activity, low motivation, and executive dysfunction. ∼

Neurotransmitters of Wakefulness

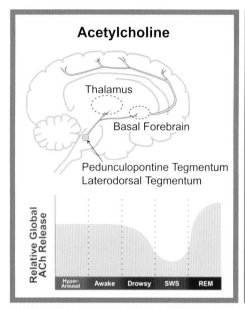

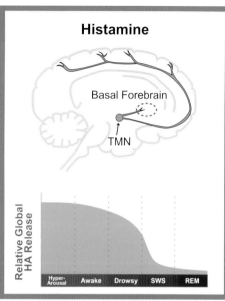

Figure 2.9 Cholinergic cells in the pedunculopontine and laterodorsal tegmentum (PPT/LDT) fire rapidly during wake and are quiet during sleep. A subpopulation of these cells resumes firing during rapid eye movement (REM) sleep. PPT/LDT neurons project to cholinergic cells in the basal forebrain and to glutamatergic cells in the thalamus to drive cortical activation.

Figure 2.10 In the brain, histamine (HA) is produced solely by cells in the TMN, and the densest histaminergic projections are to the basal forebrain and the cerebral cortex. Firing rates of TMN cells correlate with arousal level during wakefulness and completely cease during all stages of sleep.

Although overall wakefulness arises from the interaction of numerous arousal circuits, individual circuits likely mediate specific aspects of arousal. Histamine (HA) and acetylcholine (ACh) are the most important neurotransmitters for maintaining a state of wakefulness. Lesions of either the TMN or pedunculopontine and laterodorsal tegmental (PPT/LDT) nuclei produce a comatose-like chronic sleep state in animals. However, ACh is also highly elevated in the cortex during REM sleep while histaminergic circuits are virtually silent. This indicates that HA is likely more important for conscious thought processes during wakefulness, while ACh is more important for general cortical activities, such as sensory processing, that occur during both wake and REM sleep states.

Another neurotransmitter recently identified as playing a key role in arousal is hypocretin (HC, also known as orexin). When HC is administered to animals, it increases wakefulness, feeding behavior, locomotor activity, and sympathetic

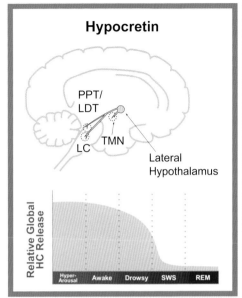

Figure 2.11 The neurotransmitter hypocretin (HC; also called orexin) is made by a small population of cells in the lateral hypothalamus (LH) that project widely, especially to key arousal loci. HC release is controlled in a circadian fashion to stabilize arousal circuits during the waking state.

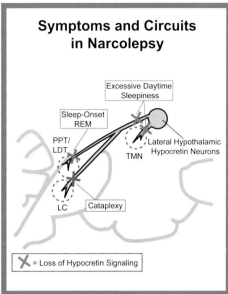

Figure 2.12 In narcolepsy, loss of HC signaling results in reduced excitation of arousal circuits, leading to excessive sleepiness and unstable sleep-/wake-state transitions. Instability in the locus coeruleus (LC) can result in abrupt loss of muscle tone, or cataplexy; similarly, instability in the PPT/LDT area can cause sudden transitions into REM sleep.

nervous system activity. HC-producing cells are limited to the LH, but they project widely to other arousal loci, especially the TMN and ARAS nuclei. The critical role of HC in mediating wakefulness was realized with the discovery that loss of HC in humans and animals leads to narcolepsy. Hypocretin is thought to stabilize wakefulness by suppressing REM sleep and lowering the activation threshold for arousal, i.e., increasing the excitatory tone of arousal circuits (Sutcliffe & de Lecea, 2002). Loss of HC signaling thus can cause inappropriate transitions into REM during waking (sleep-onset REM periods) and difficulty maintaining arousal, which leads to symptoms of excessive daytime sleepiness. In addition, cataplexy results from the reduced activity of noradrenergic locus coeruleus (LC) neurons that maintain muscle tone during arousal. These neurons are normally inhibited during REM sleep to prevent "acting out" dreams, but since patients with narcolepsy have a reduced hypocretin tone in the LC, this inhibition can improperly occur when awake. ~

Neuromodulators of Arousal

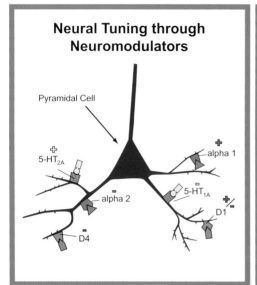

Neural Tuning through Neuromodulators

Pyramidal Cell

5-HT$_{2A}$
alpha 1
alpha 2
5-HT$_{1A}$
D1
D4

Local Regulation of Monoamine Levels

Monoamine Degradation
Monoamine Transporter

Figure 2.13 Norepinephrine (NE), serotonin (5-HT), and dopamine (DA), are neuromodulators of arousal. They can exert both excitatory and inhibitory influences on target networks through different receptors. This dual action allows neuromodulators to "tune" the response of neurons, such as the prefrontal cortical pyramidal neuron shown here.

Figure 2.14 In the PFC, the relative concentration of monoamines can create either an excitatory or inhibitory tone. NE and 5-HT reuptake transporters as well as the enzymes COMT (catechol-O-methyltransferase) and MAO (monoamine oxidase) are particularly important monoamine regulators.

The arousal circuits described so far are generally excitatory, elevating cortical activity. The monoamines play a different role in arousal, sculpting neural processing according to the internal and external environments. The monoaminergic circuits in the brain include serotonin (5-HT), norepinephrine (NE), and dopamine (DA), and affect nearly all aspects of cognition and behavior. These neurotransmitters are often referred to as neuromodulators. Their actions can be described as influencing the tone of the neuron. For example, NE acting through α_2-adrenoceptors on cortical pyramidal cells creates a negative tone such that inhibitory responses are amplified and excitatory responses are dampened. Conversely, α_1-adrenoceptor stimulation on pyramidal cells creates an excitatory tone (Gottesmann, 2002). The combination of excitatory and inhibitory influences acts to "tune" the response of the neuronal network. 5-HT and DA can modulate cortical processing in a similar manner.

In general, the release of monoamines in the brain correlates with arousal, yet the behavioral effect of elevated monoamines depends on the target network. Widespread neurotransmitter release is controlled by the firing activity of neurons, although local levels can also be controlled through activation of presynaptic

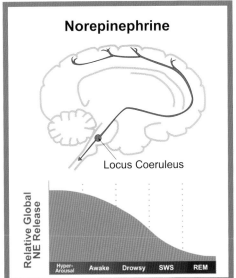

Figure 2.15 The major locus of NE-producing cells is the locus coeruleus (LC), which projects widely across the cortical mantle, as well as to motor and autonomic spinal pathways. NE modulates sensory vigilance, heightening arousal in response to salient external stimuli.

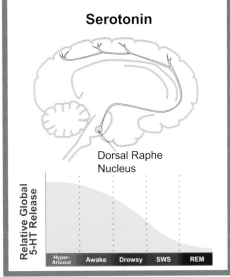

Figure 2.16 Serotonergic projections to the cerebral cortex stem largely from the dorsal raphe nucleus (DRN). The DRN receives strong input from emotion centers, especially the amygdala; thus, this circuit modulates internal and external vigilance to influence arousal based on mood and anxiety.

receptors on the axon terminal. Local control of monoamine levels is also determined by their clearance from the synapse. Monoamines can be reabsorbed by the presynaptic cell through specific transporter pumps or broken down by the enzymes monoamine oxidase (MAO) and catechol-O-methyltransferase (COMT). Drugs that act to inhibit reuptake through transporter pumps (reuptake inhibitors) or inhibit MAO or COMT generally increase behavioral arousal.

The role of each neuromodulator in arousal is related to the principal factors driving its release. The LC, which contains the majority of NE-producing neurons in the brain, receives input from sensory and visceral systems and is highly activated in response to external arousal stimuli such as loud noises or pain. Thus, the main role of NE may be to focus sensory vigilance during arousal. In addition, NE projections to the autonomic nervous system result in elevated heart rate, increased blood pressure, and sweating at higher arousal levels. 5-HT projections primarily originate in the dorsal raphe nucleus (DRN), which receives dense innervations from the LC and the amygdala. 5-HT seems to be important for modulating vigilance based on stress or mood as evidenced by the mood-elevating and anxiolytic effects of selective serotonin reuptake inhibitors (SSRIs).

Neuromodulators of Arousal (cont.)

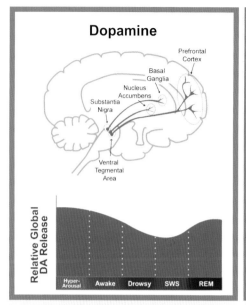

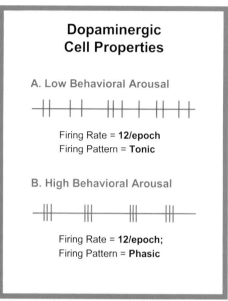

Figure 2.17 Motor activity, motivation, and cognitive behaviors are all modulated by DA circuits that originate in the ventral tegmental area (VTA) and substantia nigra (SN). DA cells receive inputs from the key areas that mediate arousal, such as the DRN, LC, and PPT/LDT, thus DA-mediated behaviors are tightly linked to arousal.

Figure 2.18 The temporal firing pattern in brainstem DA cells is modulated by arousal inputs. Tonic activity results in low DA release and is related to low arousal levels, while phasic activity releases much higher levels of DA and increases DA-mediated behaviors.

Although the firing rate of dopaminergic neurons varies very little across sleep/wake stages, recent research has uncovered the importance of firing pattern in the control of DA release. Dopaminergic neurons in the substantia nigra (SN) and ventral tegmental area (VTA) receive inputs from areas important for arousal, such as other brainstem monoaminergic nuclei, as well as descending projections from the basal forebrain. Studies in animals suggest DA release is higher during phasic burst activity, driven by arousal inputs, than during random tonic activity, which is produced internally (Floresco et al. 2003). Furthermore, the effect of DA seems to depend on the level of activity of the local neural network. During low neural activity (as in sleep or anesthesia) DA causes inhibition of the background activity, but when networks are more active, DA facilitates neural excitation in the same network (Seamans & Yang, 2004).

	Hyper-arousal	Awake	REM Sleep	SWS	Primary Role in Arousal
ACh	++	++	+++	-	Cortical Excitation
NE	+++	++	-	+	Sensory Vigilance
5-HT	+++	++	-	+	Vigilance Modulation
HA	+++	++	-	-	Conscious Awareness
HC	++	++	-	-	Arousal Stabilization
DA	+++	++	++	++	Behavior Modulation

Figure 2.19 Activity of the major arousal loci characterizes different levels of arousal. Altering the neurochemical profile of the brain with pharmacological agents influences the arousal state of the patient. Although circuits never act in isolation, general functions can be attributed to individual neurotransmitter circuits to aid the understanding of the psychopharmacology of sleep medicine.

The role of DA in arousal may be to modulate behavior based on arousal state. Indeed, the behaviors regulated by the dopaminergic system (i.e., motor control, learning, motivation, and executive function) are all influenced by arousal. Low levels of DA result in "sleepy" behavior—unfocused thought, slow movement, and low motivation.

It is the interaction of all the circuits discussed that generates the complex spectrum of arousal behaviors in humans. Individual circuits have numerous feedback loops and multiple connections with each other such that no single circuit can be altered without affecting many. However, in psychopharmacology, it is useful to understand the dominant behaviors that are related to each circuit in order to rationally select the best treatment option for patients based on their symptoms. ~

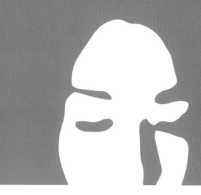

SUMMARY POINTS

- Pathways originating in the brainstem and the hypothalamus play key roles in cortical arousal for maintaining wakefulness

- There are multiple arousal circuits that interact to produce a spectrum of arousal behaviors ranging from excessive sleepiness to stimulated arousal

- NE, DA, and 5-HT from brainstem nuclei are modulatory neurotransmitters important for arousal and cognitive function; HA from the hypothalamus and ACh from the basal forebrain directly excite the cortex to maintain wakefulness

- DA release is low during sleepiness and high during wakefulness; DA may mediate arousal-related behaviors such as motor activity, motivation, and cognition

- Executive function relies on optimal arousal of the dorsolateral prefrontal cortex (DLPFC); since the DLPFC is sensitive to sleep deprivation, executive dysfunction often accompanies excessive sleepiness in sleep disorders

- In narcolepsy, arousal circuits are unstable due to a hypocretin deficiency leading to excessive sleepiness, cataplexy, and sleep-onset REM periods

SLEEP DETECTIVE

George suffers from primary hypersomnia and requires medication to treat his excessive sleepiness. His managed care provider refuses to cover the medication under the assumption that George's sleepiness does not have a biological cause. Explain to George's provider how symptoms of excessive sleepiness can arise from malfunctioning circuits in the brain.

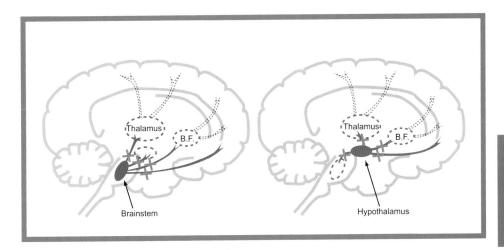

Excessive sleepiness has multiple causes. For most people, the symptom results from sleep deprivation and can be relieved by getting more sleep, but some people actually have a neurobiological malfunction, diagnosed as primary hypersomnia, that requires medical treatment. The brain depends on the coordination of multiple arousal circuits to maintain wakefulness. When any one of these circuits malfunctions, excessive sleepiness can occur. The exact cause of primary hypersomnia is unknown, but it may result from loss of cortical excitation by the ARAS, insufficient histamine signaling, or reduced cholinergic activity. Because the excessive sleepiness in primary hypersomnia is due to a biological malfunction in arousal, the best way to treat it is to use pharmacological agents that stimulate the brain's arousal circuits.

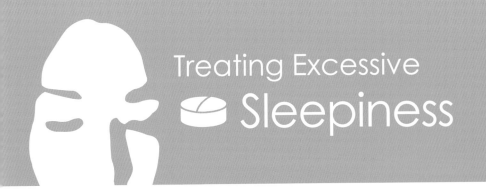

Treating Excessive Sleepiness

OBJECTIVES

- Compare the similarities and differences in brain activation and neurotransmitter release among wake-promoting drugs

- Explain how different mechanisms of action lead to different behavioral outcomes for psychostimulants, caffeine, and modafinil

- Describe the effects of wake-promoting drugs on sleep

- Assess the risks and benefits of treatment options for sleepiness in sleep disorders

- Identify drug options that may improve executive function in patients with sleep disorders or the "deficit syndrome," and specify how each improves prefrontal cortical activity

CLINICAL APPLICATIONS

Mechanisms of Action and Interaction

Understanding the psychopharmacology of wake-promoting agents leads to better individualized patient care.

Sleep Detective

Kathy finds herself falling asleep frequently and at inopportune times throughout the day. She is being treated for early-stage Parkinson's Disease with a DA agonist. What treatment options would you recommend for Kathy's sleepiness?

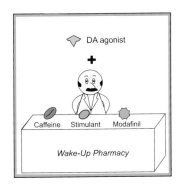

Psychopharmacology of Wakefulness

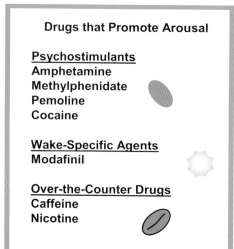

Drugs that Promote Arousal

<u>Psychostimulants</u>
Amphetamine
Methylphenidate
Pemoline
Cocaine

<u>Wake-Specific Agents</u>
Modafinil

<u>Over-the-Counter Drugs</u>
Caffeine
Nicotine

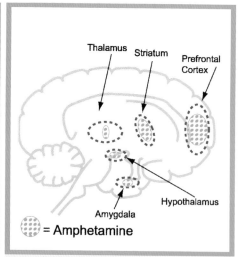

= Amphetamine

Figure 3.1 Prescription drug options for promoting wakefulness include modafinil and psychostimulants such as amphetamines and methylphenidate. Caffeine is also widely used for its arousal effects and is generally effective in overcoming symptoms of sleepiness.

Figure 3.2a This series of figures represents a model for the relative neural activation due to administration of wake-promoting drugs based on data from c-fos activation studies in rodents (Engber et al. 1998; Singewald et al. 2003). Psychostimulants cause widespread activation of regions involved in arousal, as well as motor, emotion, and reward pathways.

In order to treat excessive sleepiness in patients, it is essential to understand the pharmacological mechanisms for promoting wakefulness. This module will describe the mechanisms of action and how these mechanisms translate into a behavioral response for the primary classes of agents used to alleviate sleepiness in sleep and psychiatric disorders. When relevant, non-pharmacological treatment options will also be discussed. In many patients, excessive sleepiness can also be treated by assuring better nighttime sleep. The treatment of chronic insomnia with hypnotics or restless legs syndrome with dopamine (DA) agonists are approaches that are explored in the other books in this series.

Here we will explore the three main classes of drugs that are used principally for their arousal effects: psychostimulants; the new, non-stimulant wake-promoter, modafinil; and caffeine (a methylxanthine). Module 2 discussed the key pathways for generating arousal in the brain. Hyperarousal results from enhanced excitation of monoaminergic brainstem nuclei, while a state of calm wakefulness includes histamine (HA) activation of the cortex and moderate levels of monoamine release. Psychostimulants such as amphetamine and methylphenidate cause widespread

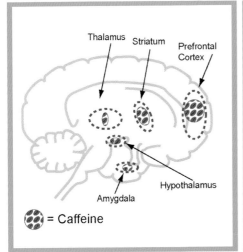

Figure 3.2b Caffeine has only a slightly more restricted pattern of activation than amphetamine, although the two agents promote arousal through different mechanisms. Since many of the same pathways are activated by caffeine and psychostimulants, they tend to share a similar profile of side effects.

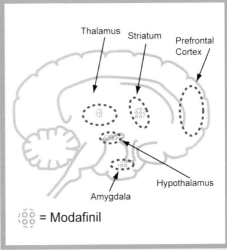

Figure 3.2c Modafinil is considered a non-stimulant, wake-promoting agent, due to its relatively limited pattern of central nervous system activation. Modafinil specifically activates neurons in wake-promoting regions such as the posterior hypothalamus, with relatively little action on reward and motor pathways.

activation of the central nervous system, and their wake-promoting actions are due largely to their effects on the monoaminergic circuits.

If caffeine were discovered today, it would likely be a controlled substance. In the brain, caffeine activates many of the same circuits as psychostimulants. For this reason, it can produce many of the same side effects as psychostimulants, such as hyperactivity, anxiety, and dependence. However, the wake-promoting benefits of caffeine are generally experienced with low doses, while many side effects do not emerge until larger doses are ingested.

The newest drug for treating excessive sleepiness is modafinil, which entered the U.S. market in 1999, for the treatment of narcolepsy. Modafinil's pattern of activation in the brain is more limited than other wake-promoting drugs, and it seems to act specifically on the HA pathway to promote calm wakefulness. At pharmacologically effective doses, there are few side effects as well as very little abuse potential. Because of the more favorable risk/benefit ratio with modafinil, it has become the first-line agent for treating many disorders of sleepiness. ~

Mechanisms of Action: Psychostimulants

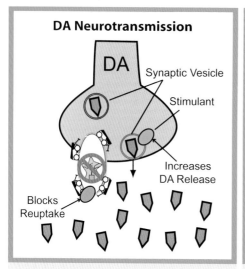

DA Neurotransmission

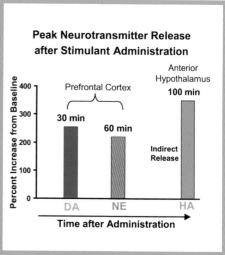

Peak Neurotransmitter Release after Stimulant Administration

Figure 3.3 Psychostimulants enhance monoamine neurotransmission by blocking monoamine reuptake and increasing neurotransmitter release. The dopaminergic system is the primary target that gives rise to the behavioral effects of psychostimulants, but norepinephrine (NE) and serotonin (5-HT) also contribute.

Figure 3.4 Dopamine (DA) and NE levels are rapidly elevated in the prefrontal cortex (PFC) after psychostimulant administration in rodents (Bymaster et al. 2002). Psychostimulants also cause the release of histamine (HA), probably through secondary mechanisms (Ito et al. 1997). The high concentrations of these neurotransmitters trigger a state of heightened arousal.

Pscyhostimulants increase synaptic levels of DA, norepinephrine (NE), and serotonin (5-HT) through simultaneously blocking reuptake transporters and increasing neurotransmitter release. In addition, they are weak monoamine oxidase (MAO) inhibitors further elevating synaptic monoamine levels. Enhanced DA neurotransmission appears to be the primary mechanism of action for stimulant drugs. Based on a large body of genetic and pharmacological studies in animals, the behavioral arousal from psychostimulants requires the activity of D_1 and D_2 receptors as well as the DA transporter (DAT). Psychostimulants act indiscriminately on DA circuits. Thus, motor, reward, and cognitive pathways are all stimulated, giving rise to hyperactivity, addiction, and in some cases of high dose abuse, thought disorder.

Elevated mood is commonly reported by people who use psychostimulants, particularly amphetamines. This behavioral effect is likely due to activation of serotonergic circuits as well as DA activation of reward circuitry. The increase in NE release from the descending locus coeruleus (LC) projections, as well as secondary epinephrine release, is largely responsible for the autonomic effects of

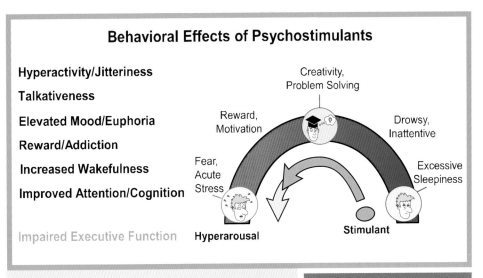

Behavioral Effects of Psychostimulants

Hyperactivity/Jitteriness

Talkativeness

Elevated Mood/Euphoria

Reward/Addiction

Increased Wakefulness

Improved Attention/Cognition

Impaired Executive Function

Creativity, Problem Solving

Reward, Motivation

Drowsy, Inattentive

Fear, Acute Stress

Excessive Sleepiness

Hyperarousal

Stimulant

Figure 3.5 Psychostimulants are effective in increasing wakefulness; however, they activate multiple arousal circuits, leading to increased arousal behaviors. High levels of DA release in the striatum augment motor activity, while DA release in the nucleus accumbens (NA) activates the reward pathway and is the reason psychostimulants have a high abuse potential.

Pharmacodynamics

	t1/2	Relative Potency
Methylphenidate	6 h	++
Amphetamine	12 h	+++
Pemoline	16 h	+

psychostimulants. Autonomic effects include elevated blood pressure, raised heart rate, pupil dilation, and sweating. HA is also released secondarily in the hypothalamus and may contribute to wakefulness through inhibiting the sleep-promoter.

Some people experience enhanced executive function with psychostimulants, but usually only if hypofunction is present, such as in attention deficit hyperactivity disorder (ADHD). Hyperstimulation of monoamine neurotransmission can cause a decline in cognitive performance, as discussed in the previous module. Extended amphetamine use in normal humans has been known to lead to cognitive and behavioral disorders. Paranoid psychosis and emotional blunting can occur after only five to ten repetitive doses of a psychostimulant. Another risk of psychostimulant use is a six-fold increase in the chance of stroke and a risk of inducing seizures. Psychostimulants, especially amphetamines, are the most effective wake-promoting agents, but their use is only warranted in difficult-to-treat cases of excessive sleepiness. Patients treated with these stimulants should be closely monitored for thought disorder and other negative side effects. ~

Mechanisms of Action: Caffeine

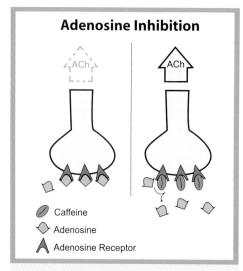

Adenosine Inhibition

Caffeine
Adenosine
Adenosine Receptor

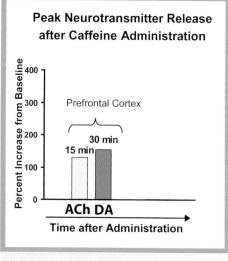

Peak Neurotransmitter Release after Caffeine Administration

Percent Increase from Baseline

Prefrontal Cortex

30 min
15 min

ACh DA

Time after Administration

Figure 3.6 The wake-promoting effects of caffeine are due to adenosine A₁ receptor antagonism. Adenosine normally inhibits arousal by decreasing cholinergic neurotransmission in the basal forebrain. Caffeine blocks this inhibition, leading to increased cortical arousal.

Figure 3.7 Caffeine acts quickly to promote acetylcholine (ACh) release in the cortex (Acquas et al. 2002). Adenosine receptor antagonism also causes local DA release in the PFC, and at higher doses, in other DA target areas.

Caffeine has a potent stimulating effect on the brain, and in high doses it produces some of the same side effects seen with psychostimulant use. The wake-promoting action of caffeine and other methylxanthines is through inhibition of the brain's endogenous sleep homeostatic mechanism, adenosine. Adenosine is sedative in nature, promoting a decline in arousal through adenosine A_1 receptor-mediated hyperpolarization of cholinergic cells in the basal forebrain.

As an A_1 receptor antagonist, caffeine blocks the effects of adenosine, effectively elevating cortical acetylcholine (ACh) levels. ACh is implicated in global cortical activation and attention; likewise, caffeine produces general arousal effects and enhanced performance on attention tasks. There is evidence that these effects from caffeine are more pronounced in sleep-deprived individuals than well-rested ones, which suggests caffeine acts by boosting normal wakefulness rather than stimulating hyperarousal.

DA release is also stimulated by caffeine. Adenosine A_1 and A_{2A} receptors often colocalize with D_1 and D_2 receptors, respectively. Thus, caffeine may increase

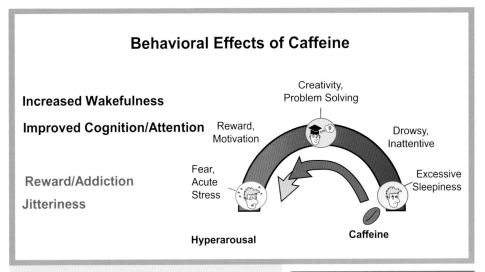

Figure 3.8 In moderate doses, wakefulness is the main effect of caffeine. However, higher doses can cause jitteriness, and repeated intake can lead to caffeine addiction. These side effects are attributed to further activation of arousal behaviors due to local increase of DA in the striatum and the NA.

Pharmacodynamics

Peak plasma levels= 30–75 min
$t_{1/2}$ = 3–7 h
(depends on age, gender, smoking, oral contraceptive use)

DA through A_1 receptor antagonism in the prefrontal cortex (PFC) and nucleus accumbens (NA) and by antagonizing adenosine A_{2A} receptors in striatal dopaminergic areas. Although DA is responsible for the stimulant-like side effects experienced with caffeine intake, animal studies suggest that it is not required for the wake-promoting effects.

Jitteriness and hyperactivity are common side effects of striatal DA stimulation that occur with higher caffeine doses. Many coffee drinkers describe a mild "buzz" with caffeine use that probably results from activation of dopaminergic reward circuitry. In addition, patients who consume more than 300 or 400 mg of caffeine per day (there is 100–150 mg of caffeine in one cup of coffee) may experience withdrawal symptoms, especially headache and fatigue, if they abruptly stop caffeine use. Long-term use of caffeine has been linked to gastrointestinal disturbances, making it intolerable as a treatment for excessive sleepiness in most patients with chronic sleep disorders. However, intermittent use may be beneficial for people who experience transient sleepiness, such as rotating-shift workers. ～

Mechanisms of Action: Modafinil

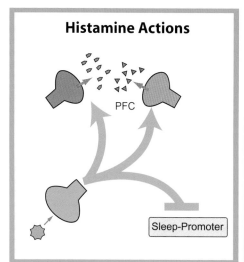

Figure 3.9 Modafinil's mechanism of action is still largely unknown. Animal studies have found that cells in the posterior hypothalamus are preferentially activated with modafinil administration, and this likely leads to the observed increase in HA release. HA can stimulate DA and NE release in the cortex.

Figure 3.10 HA is probably the primary neurotransmitter mediating the effects of modafinil. HA release happens gradually, peaking around four hours after modafinil administration (Ishizuka et al. 2003). NE and DA levels are also elevated in the PFC, although this is likely secondary to HA release (de Saint-Hilaire et al. 2001).

The precise mechanism of action for modafinil remains unknown, but a growing body of evidence points to the histaminergic system. Modafinil produces a state of calm wakefulness, linked to the hypothalamic-cortical circuit, rather than stimulated arousal. Modafinil administration in animals activates cells in the posterior hypothalamus, including hypocretin- and HA-producing neurons. Because modafinil is effective in people with narcolepsy who lack hypocretin function, HA is considered the primary neurotransmitter involved in the wake-promoting effects of modafinil.

The role of HA in arousal has long been known due to the sedating effects of antihistamines. It is thus not surprising that a drug that enhances HA function would have arousal effects. HA can excite cortical neurons and inhibit neurons in the sleep-promoting ventrolateral preoptic (VLPO) area in the hypothalamus. HA can also facilitate the release of other monoamines in the cortex, such as DA and NE; however, monoamine release from subcortical areas is unaffected by HA or modafinil. This limited activation pattern explains why modafinil has few autonomic effects and does not induce hyperarousal behaviors.

Behavioral Effects of Modafinil

Increased Wakefulness

Improved Cognition/Attention

Enhanced Executive Function

Creativity,
Problem Solving

Reward,
Motivation

Drowsy,
Inattentive

Fear,
Acute
Stress

Excessive
Sleepiness

Hyperarousal

Modafinil

Figure 3.11 The relatively specific action of modafinil on histaminergic circuits leads to few behavioral effects other than wakefulness. Local, moderate monoamine release in the PFC with modafinil may enhance executive function, but modafinil acts very little on other monoamine circuits, so hyperarousal behaviors are not stimulated.

Pharmacodynamics

Steady state levels reached after 2–4 days

$t_{1/2}$ = 15 h

Peak plasma levels: 2–4 h

There are conflicting studies regarding the role of DA in the wake-promoting effects of modafinil. Modafinil binds to the dopamine transporter (DAT) with an affinity similar to amphetamines (although much weaker than cocaine or bupropion), and DAT knockout mice lack the normal behavioral arousal response to modafinil. On the other hand, modafinil remains effective in the presence of the D_1/D_2 receptor antagonist, haloperidol, suggesting DA signaling through these receptors is not necessary to promote wakefulness.

Several studies have shown enhanced executive function with modafinil during sleep deprivation and in patients with arousal deficits (narcolepsy, obstructive sleep apnea [OSA], shift-work sleep disorder, and ADHD). Unlike psychostimulants and caffeine, modafinil has few motor side effects and so far, studies have not found a significant incidence of tolerance or dependence. These characteristics have pushed modafinil to the forefront of treatment options for excessive sleepiness, especially in patients with a history of drug abuse or sensitivity to stimulants. ~

Comparing Wake-Promoting Drugs

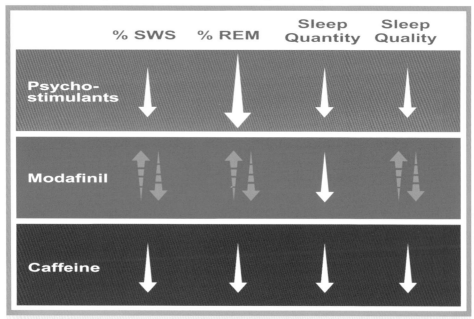

Figure 3.12 All wake-promoting drugs decrease sleep quantity, but they differ in their effect on sleep architecture and sleep quality. Caffeine moderately decreases slow wave sleep (SWS) and rapid eye movement (REM) sleep and causes sleep disruption, but only if taken within several hours of sleep. Psychostimulants dramatically reduce the amount of REM and cause sleep fragmentation. Current data suggests the effects of modafinil on sleep quality and architecture are mild.

There is concern about the effects of wake-promoting drugs on consequent sleep, especially in patients with sleep disorders. Amphetamines and methylphenidate cause a dramatic reduction in REM sleep as well as sleep fragmentation and insomnia, which can exacerbate sleepiness symptoms (Qureshi and Lee-Chiong, 2004). Caffeine also decreases REM sleep as well as deep SWS in favor of lighter sleep stages, and it causes rapid cycling between sleep stages (Boutrel and Koob, 2004). Because caffeine has a short half-life though, the effects on sleep are only seen when consumed within several hours of sleep onset. The data on the impact of modafinil on sleep are limited. In humans, rebound sleep quality and quantity are unaffected by modafinil after prolonged sleep deprivation (Buguet et al. 1995), but further research is still needed.

One limitation of all wake-promoting drugs in treating excessive sleepiness is that the wake-promoting effects tend not to last all day, creating a dilemma over whether to use supplemental drug doses later in the day and risk disrupting sleep, or to suffer with sleepiness through the latter part of the day. A new version of modafinil, termed armodafinil (the 'R' enantiomer of the drug) has a longer half-

	Psycho-stimulants	Caffeine	Modafinil
Efficacy	Good	Good	Good
Common Side Effects	Nervousness, Headaches, Insomnia, Anorexia, GI Disturbances, Mood Changes, Hyperactivity	Nervousness, Headaches, Insomnia, Anorexia, GI Disturbances, Mood Changes, Hyperactivity	Headache, Nausea, Dry Mouth, Insomnia, Hyperactivity
Tolerance	Yes	Can Develop	Very Little
Dependence	High Potential	Moderate Potential	Low Potential

Figure 3.13 While all of the wake-promoting agents discussed are good at stimulating arousal, they differ in side effects, tolerance, and dependence. This chart compares the psychostimulants, caffeine, and modafinil, based on the wealth of data in humans reported so far. The side effect profile of each drug relates to the areas of activation shown at the beginning of this module.

FDA-Approved Uses for Wake-Promoting Drugs
Amphetamines
ADHD
Narcolepsy
Weight loss
Methylphenidate
ADHD
Narcolepsy
Modafinil
Obstructive sleep apnea
Shift-work sleep disorder
Narcolepsy

life than its predecessor, but a similar safety profile. In clinical trials, armodafinil helped patients with narcolepsy, shift-work sleep disorder, and OSA maintain wakefulness for longer periods, yet without disrupting subsequent sleep (data on file, Cephalon, Inc.).

In general, amphetamines are the most potent drugs for promoting wakefulness, though their use carries substantial risks. One "head-to-head" study suggests that modafinil and caffeine tend to be equally effective in maintaining wakefulness caused by sleep deprivation in humans (Wesensten, 2002). Cost and availability may limit the use of modafinil since generic psychostimulants and caffeine are generally less expensive and more widely available. Although caffeine, psychostimulants, and modafinil are all effective in promoting wakefulness, individual patients may respond better to, or be less tolerant of, certain agents compared with others. The clinician must choose an appropriate treatment based on their understanding of how each drug works in relation to the symptoms and medical history of the patient. ～

Treatment Guidelines: Obstructive Sleep Apnea

CPAP Therapy

Indication: First-line treatment for obstructive sleep apnea.

Action: Reduce airway obstruction by delivering continuous air pressure

Benefit: Eliminate apnea disturbance, reverse functional impairment

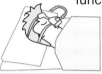

Surgical Therapy

Indication: Obvious upper airway obstruction, limited benefit from other options

Action: Remove upper airway obstruction

Benefit: Eliminate apnea disturbance, reverse functional impairment

Figure 3.14 Continuous positive airway pressure (CPAP) is generally the first-line treatment for OSA. While functional outcomes are very good with CPAP, patient compliance can be a problem due to the inconvenience of the apparatus and a lack of perceived benefit.

Figure 3.15 There are several surgical methods available for removing the upper airway obstruction in OSA. These treatments are highly effective, with 60–90% of patients experiencing a reversal of symptoms (Riley et al. 2000).

While there is no question that patients with OSA need treatment for their own safety and that of others, the question of how best to treat these patients is more difficult. Continuous positive airway pressure (CPAP) was developed in the 1980s to treat nighttime breathing difficulties. When used regularly, it is extremely effective in reducing apnea events and increasing the quality of life for patients. However, the equipment can be uncomfortable and many patients are resistant to using it, especially if they do not recognize the risks associated with chronic sleepiness. In addition, patients using CPAP may experience nasal congestion or sinus and chest discomfort related to the therapy. Long-term compliance with CPAP treatment is reported to be around 65–80%. In many cases, the patient's perception of improvement correlates with compliance. In non-compliant patients, therefore, it may be useful to provide an adjunct dose of modafinil to improve daytime functioning. Modafinil is currently the best-documented and the only FDA-approved drug for treating residual sleepiness in patients concurrently using CPAP therapy. It is important that modafinil not be the sole therapeutic agent for sleep apnea since it does not eliminate apnea events and therefore leaves the patient at risk for hypoxic-induced brain damage. Because of the potential risks associated

Pharmacotherapy

Indication:
Residual daytime sleepiness,
CPAP and surgery are not options

Action:
Improve daytime arousal
- **Modafinil: 100–400mg once/day**
  May reduce apnea events
- **Protriptyline: 10 mg (+/-) twice/day**
- **HRT in postmenopausal women**

Benefit:
Reduce daytime sleepiness,
Decrease functional impairment

Weight Loss for Treating Obstructive Sleep Apnea

Change in apnea frequency during dietary weight reduction program in a single patient

(data from Browman, et al. 1984)

Figure 3.16 Pharmacotherapy is helpful in treating residual sleepiness during CPAP therapy and may improve patient compliance. Modafinil has recently received FDA approval for treating sleepiness in OSA based on positive clinical trials in patients concurrently using CPAP. The data for the benefits of protriptyline and hormone replacement therapy (HRT) are more limited, and these drugs should only be considered as a last resort.

with psychostimulants, they are only recommended for severe, treatment-resistant sleepiness in OSA.

For patients who cannot or will not tolerate CPAP, surgery is another option. The best candidates for surgical treatment are those in whom a specific upper airway abnormality is found. In children with sleep-related breathing problems, enlarged tonsils or adenoids are common. Surgical removal of these structures will usually eliminate nighttime breathing abnormalities and also improve related attention and behavioral problems. Gastric bypass for weight loss is currently being reviewed as a possible treatment option for obese patients with OSA.

There are mixed reports on the usefulness of pharmacotherapy for reducing apnea events in patients. Protriptyline is a tricyclic antidepressant which may help reduce apnea in some patients; however, a large percentage of patients cannot tolerate its anticholinergic side effects. This drug is not FDA approved for treating OSA and should only be tried as a last resort. There are data to suggest postmenopausal women with OSA may experience substantial benefits with hormone replacement therapy, specifically estrogens. ~

Treatment Guidelines: Hypersomnia

Pharmacotherapy

Indication: Excessive daytime sleepiness

Action: Promote wakefulness
- Modafinil 100–200 mg in AM
+100–200 mg midday*
- Methylphenidate 5–20mg in AM
+5 mg midday and afternoon*
- d-amphetamine 15 mg in AM
+5 mg midday and afternoon*

Benefit: Improve daytime performance, reduce chance of accidents

(*if needed)

Pharmacotherapy

Indication: Cataplexy

Action: Reduce muscle atonia (NRI action)
- Clomipramine* 75–125 mg/day
- Viloxazine* 150–200 mg/day
- Imipramine* 75–125 mg/day
- Fluoxetine* 20–60 mg/day
- Venlafaxine* 150–300 mg/day
- Sodium oxybate 6–9 g/day

Benefit: Eliminate cataplectic attacks

Figure 3.17 Modafinil or psychostimulants can be used to reduce excessive daytime sleepiness (EDS) associated with narcolepsy or other hypersomnia disorders. Dosing should start in the morning with midday supplemental doses if needed.

Figure 3.18 Most effective anticataplectic drugs block 5-HT and NE reuptake, although no drugs in this class are currently approved by the FDA to treat cataplexy. The mechanism for sodium oxybate, the only FDA-approved treatment, is poorly characterized but may act on GABA$_B$ receptors.

Excessive daytime sleepiness (EDS) as a symptom of narcolepsy and primary hypersomnia is currently treated with wake-promoting drugs. Although research is underway, there are no alternative treatment options at present. Amphetamines are generally the most effective drug for stimulating arousal, but they have a high risk of unwanted side effects. Modafinil has become increasingly popular in treating narcolepsy and is a good choice when initiating therapy due to its excellent safety profile. Whichever agent is chosen, patients should start on a relatively high dose in the morning, so as not to disrupt nighttime sleep. If needed, small doses can be taken after midday and afternoon naps to sustain wakefulness. Methylphenidate and amphetamines are most potent when taken on an empty stomach.

Additional pharmacotherapy may be needed for patients with narcolepsy who suffer cataplexy. Most of the drugs that are effective in reducing cataplexy are antidepressants that block 5-HT or NE reuptake or have an active norepinephrine reuptake blocking metabolite. Clomipramine and fluoxetine are usually recommended as first-line agents for cataplexy. Clomipramine may also reduce symptoms of sleep paralysis and hypnagogic hallucinations, possibly related to

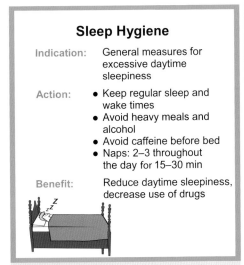

Sleep Hygiene

Indication:	General measures for excessive daytime sleepiness
Action:	• Keep regular sleep and wake times • Avoid heavy meals and alcohol • Avoid caffeine before bed • Naps: 2–3 throughout the day for 15–30 min
Benefit:	Reduce daytime sleepiness, decrease use of drugs

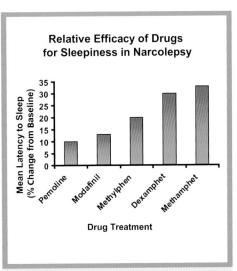

Relative Efficacy of Drugs for Sleepiness in Narcolepsy

Mean Latency to Sleep (% Change from Baseline)

Drug Treatment: Pemoline, Modafinil, Methylphen, Dexamphet, Methamphet

Figure 3.19 Good sleep hygiene is especially important for patients with hypersomnia. Napping can help maintain alertness and avoid unintentional sleep. Wake-promoting drugs should be scheduled around planned naps.

Figure 3.20 This chart compares the efficacy of many psychostimulants and modafinil in improving wakefulness in narcolepsy. Amphetamines are generally the most potent, but their side effects may make them undesirable for use in many patients (data from Mitler & Hajdukovic, 1991).

its anticholinergic properties. Sodium oxybate (GHB) is a CNS depressant and the only FDA-approved drug for treating cataplexy. There are endogenous GHB receptors in the brain, and GHB seems to have $GABA_B$ receptor agonist properties, but the drug's mechanism for reducing cataplexy is still unknown. GHB may also be effective in reducing EDS, allowing for lower doses of stimulant treatment in some patients.

Pharmacological management of other hypersomnias is generally similar to that of EDS in narcolepsy. If hypersomnia is associated with another disorder such as depression, choosing an antidepressant that reduces sleep, such as fluoxetine, may help diminish the need for additional stimulant treatment.

Behavioral measures are very important in managing EDS in sleep disorders. It is important that patients adhere to good sleep hygiene guidelines. Naps in particular have proven to be very helpful in reducing the number of unwanted sleep episodes in patients with narcolepsy, as well as in maintaining a higher level of functioning throughout the day. Naps should be brief (less than 45 minutes) and regularly scheduled. ～

Targeting Executive Function

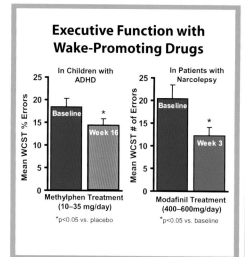

Executive Function with Wake-Promoting Drugs

In Children with ADHD

Mean WCST % Errors

Baseline
Week 16
*

Methylphen Treatment
(10–35 mg/day)
*p<0.05 vs. placebo

In Patients with Narcolepsy

Mean WCST # of Errors

Baseline
Week 3
*

Modafinil Treatment
(400–600mg/day)
*p<0.05 vs. baseline

Pharmacotherapy

Indication: Executive dysfunction in sleep disorders

Action: Enhance prefrontal cortical acitivity
• **Monoamine reuptake inhibitors: alone or adjunct with modafinil**

Benefit: Improve cognition and concentration

SRI
Serotonin Reuptake Inhibitor

NRI
Norepinephrine Reuptake Inhibitor

DRI
Dopamine Reuptake Inhibitor

Figure 3.21 In many patients, executive dysfunction associated with sleepiness will be reversed with wake-promoting drugs. Improvement in executive function, measured by the Wisconsin Card Sorting Task (WCST), can be seen with modafinil in narcolepsy patients (Schwatz et al. 2004) or methylphenidate in children with ADHD (Yang et al. 2004).

Figure 3.22 However, in some patients, residual problems of executive function may require additional treatment. Monoamine reuptake inhibitors may improve cognitive symptoms in patients with sleep disorders. (These drugs have not been FDA approved for use in sleep disorders).

Wake-promoting drugs do not provide the same benefit to all patients. Some patients will have improved cognition related to restored arousal circuits, but others may experience residual symptoms of "deficit syndrome" or a worsening of cognitive symptoms due to continued hypofunction in the PFC. For these patients, alternative pharmacological agents may be needed.

Since the cognitive problems associated with "deficit syndrome" tend to involve frontal cortical circuits, drugs that target neurotransmission important for these circuits are used to treat these problems. The monoamines, NE, DA, and 5-HT, are particularly important for tuning prefrontal cortical networks. There are currently many different drugs available that target monoamines, and most of them are antidepressants that specifically inhibit reuptake transporters. Many monoamine reuptake inhibitors appear to enhance wakefulness and are reasonable options for treating executive dysfunction in patients with sleep disorders. Tricyclic antidepressants also target monoamines, but they are not recommended for

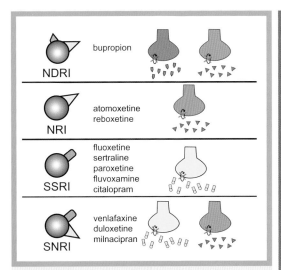

Figure 3.23 Monoamine reuptake inhibitors work by blocking a single monoamine transporter or may have multiple reuptake blocking actions. These drugs treat symptoms of the "deficit syndrome" by elevating cortical monoamine levels.

New Horizons in Drug Therapy

H₃ Receptors
- Modulate release of ACh, DA, NE, and especially HA
- Antagonists improve cognitive performance and promote wakefulness in rodents

Catechol-O-methyltransferase (COMT) Enzyme
- Inactivates DA and NE; especially important in PFC
- Inhibitors improve working memory in rodents

Nicotinic Cholinergic Receptors
- Modulate release of ACh, DA, NE, 5-HT, GABA, and glutamate
- Nicotine improves working memory in rodent models
- Nicotine improves cognition in Alzheimer's Disease, ADHD, and schizophrenia

Armodafinil
- Active enantiomer of modafinil
- All-day, wake-promoting action in human clinical trials

treating executive dysfunction related to sleepiness because they can have undesirable side effects due to their anticholinergic properties, and often they will induce sedation due to their antihistaminergic properties.

For patients with symptoms of the "deficit syndrome" related to a psychiatric disorder, modafinil can be used to treat fatigue and executive dysfunction in place of, or in addition to, other drugs. Modafinil has been shown to enhance performance on tasks of executive function in both normal, sleep-deprived adults and in those with cognitive deficits related to psychiatric disorders, such as attention deficit disorder and depression.

To improve functional outcomes for patients with sleep disorders or sleepiness related to other disorders, it is crucial to understand how drugs work and how these actions lead to behavioral responses. By knowing the circuits and neurotransmitters underlying the symptoms and treatments of various disorders, physicians can better match different treatment options to the individual symptoms of their patients. ～

Targeting Executive Function (cont.)

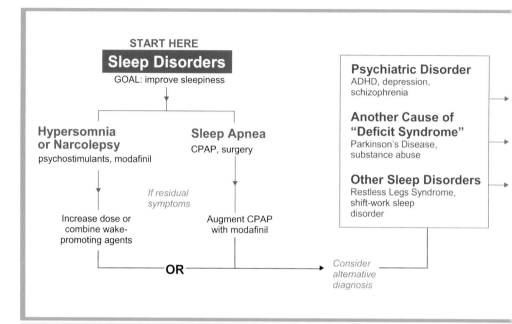

Figure 3.24 This flow chart suggests a treatment plan for patients with the "deficit syndrome." When beginning treatment of a patient with symptoms of the "deficit syndrome," first consider the primary cause of the symptoms: does the patient's history indicate a psychiatric disorder, a sleep disorder, another medical condition, or is the cause undetermined? The primary

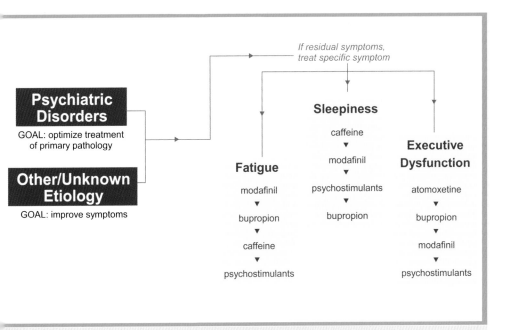

cause should be treated first. If there are residual symptoms after treatment, alternative or adjunctive options should be considered and alternative diagnoses should be explored. If there is no known cause of the patient's "deficit syndrome," the specific symptom(s) should still be treated.

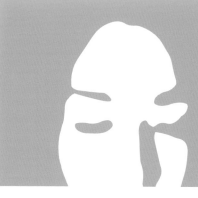

SUMMARY POINTS

- Psychostimulants (e.g., amphetamines, methylphenidate) promote arousal and are most efficacious in narcolepsy, but they have a high risk of abuse and hyperactivity due to their activation of multiple neural circuits, especially DA pathways

- Caffeine promotes general cortical arousal through enhancing cholinergic neurotransmission in the basal forebrain projections

- Modafinil works more specifically on wakefulness circuits (through HA release) and has fewer side effects than caffeine and stimulants

- OSA can be treated by CPAP or surgery; modafinil may be useful as an adjunctive therapy for residual sleepiness

- Sleepiness in narcolepsy and other hypersomnias is best treated by a combination of good sleep hygiene (including regular naps) and pharmacotherapy; modafinil or psychostimulants should be dosed throughout the day

- In patients where executive dysfunction is a problem, augmenting treatment with drugs that enhance activity in the PFC should be considered

ρ SLEEP DETECTIVE

Kathy finds herself falling asleep frequently and at inopportune times throughout the day. She is being treated for early stage Parkinson's Disease with a DA agonist. What treatment options would you recommend for Kathy's sleepiness?

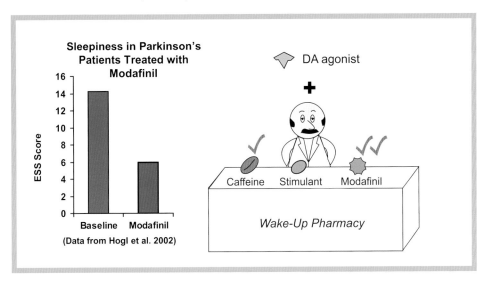

Parkinson's Disease is a progressive degeneration of DA-producing neurons from the substantia nigra and eventually, the ventral tegmental area. The DA agonist Kathy is taking to treat her disease will flood the DA receptors throughout her brain. Psychostimulants would not be a wise first choice for increasing arousal, since their primary mechanism of promoting wakefulness is through increasing synaptic DA levels. In Kathy's case, DA receptors are likely, optimally stimulated by her current therapy, and further increasing DA levels will probably not help. In fact, psychostimulants could induce motor dyskinesia and may also trigger hallucinations through their actions on subcortical DA circuits.

Modafinil is a reasonable option to treat Kathy's sleepiness. Since modafinil promotes wakefulness mainly through HA, it is more likely to be effective in her. However, there is still controversy over the role of DA in the effectiveness of modafinil. Alternatively, you could recommend that Kathy take small, regularly spaced doses of caffeine throughout the day. Caffeine maintains wakefulness independent of DA function and is very likely to help Kathy stay alert.

Abbreviations

ARAS	Ascending Reticular Activating System
ATP	Adenosine Triphosphate
CNS	Central Nervous System
COMT	catechol-O-methyltransferase
CPAP	Continuous Positive Airway Pressure
DA	Dopamine
DAT	Dopamine Transporter
DLPFC	Dorsolateral Prefrontal Cortex
DRN	Dorsal Raphe Nucleus
EDS	Excessive Daytime Sleepiness
EEG	Electroencephalography
FDA	Food and Drug Administration
GABA	Gamma-aminobutyric Acid
GHB	Sodium Oxybate
HA	Histamine
HC	Hypocretin (a.k.a. Orexin)
HLA	Human Leukocyte Antigen
HRT	Hormone Replacement Therapy
LC	Locus Coeruleus
LDT	Laterodorsal Tegmentum
LH	Lateral Hypothalamus
MAO	Monoamine Oxidase
MSLT	Multiple Sleep Latencies Test
NA	Nucleus Accumbens
NDRI	Norepinephrine and Dopamine Reuptake Inhibitor
NE	Norepinephrine (a.k.a. Noradrenaline)
NRI	Norepinephrine Reuptake Inhibitor
OSA	Obstructive Sleep Apnea
PFC	Prefrontal Cortex
PPT	Pedunculopontine Tegmentum
RDI	Respiratory Disturbance Index
REM	Rapid Eye Movement
SN	Substantia Nigra
SNRI	Serotonin and Norepinephrine Reuptake Inhibitor
SOREMPs	Sleep-Onset REM Periods
SSRI	Selective Serotonin Reuptake Inhibitor
SWS	Slow Wave Sleep
TMN	Tuberomammillary Nucleus
VAS	Visual Analog Scale
VLPO	Ventrolateral Preoptic Nucleus
VTA	Ventral Tegmental Area
WCST	Wisconsin Card Sorting Task

Appendix

Example Sleep Health Questionnaire

Sleep Hygiene Questions:

Do you go to bed at a regular time every night? Yes _____ No _____ What time? _____

Do you wake up at a regular time every day? Yes _____ No _____ What time? _____

On the average, how many hours do you spend in your bed each night? _____

On the average, how many hours do you sleep each night? _____

How long does it normally take for you to fall asleep after bedtime? _____

While in bed, do you read? Yes _____ No _____ and/or watch TV? Yes _____ No _____

Do you take naps? Yes _____ No _____ If so, what times? _____ For how long? _____

Do you smoke? Yes _____ No _____ How much? _____

How long have you been smoking? _____

Do you drink alcohol? Yes _____ No _____ What/ how much/ how often/ time of day? _____

Do you consume caffeine? Yes __ No __ What/ how much/ how often/ time of day? _____

General Sleep Problems Assessment:

Do you have difficulty falling or staying asleep? Yes_____ No _____

Please specify. _____
_____

Do you have difficulty sleeping away from home? Yes _____ No _____

Does chronic pain interfere with your sleep? Yes_____ No _____

On a scale of 1–10, 10 being most severe, rate your pain: _____

Why do you have pain?_____
_____

Do you have Gastroesophageal Reflux Disorder (GERD)? Y/N

      Hypertension (high blood pressure)? Y/N

      Chronic Obstructive Pulmonary Disease? Y/N

      Asthma? Y/N

      Diabetes? Y/N

      Depression? Y/N

Do you have any drug allergies? _____

Do you have leg jerks at night? Yes _____ No _____

Do you have daytime sleepiness? Yes _____ No _____

and/or fatigue? Yes _____ No _____

Do you have morning headaches? Yes _____ No _____

Do you have night sweats? Yes _____ No _____

Sleep Apnea Questions

Has anyone observed you snoring? Yes _____ No _____ Not Sure _____

If yes, do you snore every night? Yes _____ No _____ Not Sure _____

On a scale of 1–10, 10 being the loudest, how loudly do you snore? _____

Has anyone observed you having pauses in your breathing at night? Yes _____ No _____

How long do these pauses last? _____ How long has this occurred? _____

Do you have shortness of breath at night? Yes _____ No _____

Do you wake with a sore throat? Y/N Dry mouth? Y/N Nasal congestion ? Y/N

Has your bed partner been forced into another room because of your snoring? Yes _____ No _____

Have you experienced impotence or decreased libido? Yes _____ No _____

Do you have difficulty driving due to your sleepiness? Yes _____ No _____

Have you ever fallen asleep while driving? Yes _____ No _____ How many times? _____

Is your weight stable? Yes _____ No _____

Have you gained weight _____ or lost weight _____? # of pounds _____

Over what course of time? _____

Has your nose ever been broken? Yes _____ No _____

How and when? _____

Do you have a deviated septum? Yes _____ No _____

Have your tonsils been removed? Yes _____ No _____

Have your adenoids been removed? Yes _____ No _____

Have you had surgery to remove the uvula (UPPP)? Yes _____ No _____

Have you had any other nasal or throat surgery? Yes _____ No _____

Explain _____

_____

Narcolepsy Questions:

Do you have hallucinations while falling asleep or upon awakening? Yes _____ No _____

Do you ever have sudden unexplained, involuntary, or inappropriate sleep attacks?

Yes _____ No _____

Do you dream during these attacks? Yes _____ No _____

Do you have total body paralysis while falling asleep or upon awakening?

Yes _____ No _____

Do you have severe muscular weakness elicited by strong emotions (cataplexy)?

Yes _____ No _____

Example Sleep Diary

	Sleep-wake Schedule	/ /2005	/ /2005	/ /2005
Complete this section when you wake up	What time did you go to bed?	__:__AM/PM	__:__AM/PM	__:__AM/PM
	How long did it take you to fall asleep?			
	How many times did you wake up from your sleep?			
	What time did you wake up?	__:__AM/PM	__:__AM/PM	__:__AM/PM
	How refreshed did you feel when you woke up? Rate on a scale of 1-5 (1=fatigued; 5=refreshed)	1 2 3 4 5	1 2 3 4 5	1 2 3 4 5
	How many hours did you sleep?			
Complete this section before you go to bed	**During the day did you:**			
	Consume caffeine? Time(s) of day?	Y / N	Y / N	Y / N
	Exercise? Time of day? How long?	Y / N	Y / N	Y / N
	Drink alcohol? Time(s) of day?	Y / N	Y / N	Y / N
	Take medications? Name? Time of day?	Y / N	Y / N	Y / N

/ /2005	/ /2005	/ /2005	/ /2005
__:__AM/PM	__:__AM/PM	__:__AM/PM	__:__AM/PM
__:__AM/PM	__:__AM/PM	__:__AM/PM	__:__AM/PM
1 2 3 4 5	1 2 3 4 5	1 2 3 4 5	1 2 3 4 5
Y / N	Y / N	Y / N	Y / N
Y / N	Y / N	Y / N	Y / N
Y / N	Y / N	Y / N	Y / N
Y / N	Y / N	Y / N	Y / N

Reference List

Acquas E, Tanda G, Di CG. Differential effects of caffeine on dopamine and acetylcholine transmission in brain areas of drug-naive and caffeine-pretreated rats. Neuropsychopharmacology 2002;27(2):182-193.

Baguet JP, Hammer L, Levy P, Pierre H, Rossini E, Mouret S et al. Night-time and diastolic hypertension are common and underestimated conditions in newly diagnosed apnoeic patients. J Hypertens 2005;23(3):521-527.

Basheer R, Strecker RE, Thakkar MM, McCarley RW. Adenosine and sleep-wake regulation. Prog Neurobiol 2004;73(6):379-396.

Bassetti C, Gugger M, Bischof M, Mathis J, Sturzenegger C, Werth E et al. The narcoleptic borderland: a multimodal diagnostic approach including cerebrospinal fluid levels of hypocretin-1 (orexin A). Sleep Medicine 2003;4(1): 7-12.

Bassiri AG, Guilleminault C. Clinical Features and Evaluation of Obstructive Sleep Apnea-Hypopnea Syndrome. In: Kyger MH, Dement WC, Roth T, editors. Sleep Medicine. 3rd ed Saunders; 2000. p. 869-878.

Boutrel B, Koob GF. What keeps us awake: the neuropharmacology of stimulants and wakefulness-promoting medications. Sleep 2004;27(6):1181-1194.

Buguet A, Montmayeur A, Pigeau R, Naitoh P. Modafinil, d-amphetamine and placebo during 64 hours of sustained mental work. II. Effects on two nights of recovery sleep. J Sleep Res 1995;4(4):229-241.

Bymaster FP, Katner JS, Nelson DL, Hemrick-Luecke SK, Threlkeld PG, Heiligenstein JH et al. Atomoxetine increases extracellular levels of norepinephrine and dopamine in prefrontal cortex of rat: a potential mechanism for efficacy in attention deficit/hyperactivity disorder. Neuropsychopharmacology 2002;27(5):699-711.

Chervin RD, Archbold KH, Dillon JE, Panahi P, Pituch KJ, Dahl RE et al. Inattention, hyperactivity, and symptoms of sleep-disordered breathing. Pediatrics 2002;109(3):449-456.

Dawson D, Reid K. Fatigue, alcohol and performance impairment. Nature 1997;388(6639):235.

de Saint HZ, Orosco M, Rouch C, Blanc G, Nicolaidis S. Variations in extracellular monoamines in the prefrontal cortex and medial hypothalamus after modafinil administration: a microdialysis study in rats. Neuroreport 2001;12(16):3533-3537.

Engber TM, Koury EJ, Dennis SA, Miller MS, Contreras PC, Bhat RV. Differential patterns of regional c-Fos induction in the rat brain by amphetamine and the novel wakefulness-promoting agent modafinil. Neurosci Lett 1998;241(2-3): 95-98.

Floresco SB, West AR, Ash B, Moore H, Grace AA. Afferent modulation of dopamine neuron firing differentially regulates tonic and phasic dopamine transmission. Nat Neurosci 2003;6(9):968-973.

Fulda S, Schulz H. Cognitive dysfunction in sleep disorders. Sleep Med Rev 2001;5(6):423-445.

Gencik M, Dahmen N, Wieczorek S, Kasten M, Bierbrauer J, Anghelescu I et al. A prepro-orexin gene polymorphism is associated with narcolepsy. Neurology 2001;56(1):115-117.

George CF. Reduction in motor vehicle collisions following treatment of sleep apnoea with nasal CPAP. Thorax 2001;56(7):508-512.

Gottesmann C. The neurochemistry of waking and sleeping mental activity: the disinhibition-dopamine hypothesis. Psychiatry Clin Neurosci 2002;56(4): 345-354.

Hogl B, Saletu M, Brandauer E, Glatzl S, Frauscher B, Seppi K et al. Modafinil for the treatment of daytime sleepiness in Parkinson's disease: a double-blind, randomized, crossover, placebo-controlled polygraphic trial. Sleep 2002;25(8): 905-909.

Ishizuka T, Sakamoto Y, Sakurai T, Yamatodani A. Modafinil increases histamine release in the anterior hypothalamus of rats. Neurosci Lett 2003;339(2):143-146.

Ito C, Onodera K, Yamatodani A, Watanabe T, Sato M. The effect of methamphetamine on histamine release in the rat hypothalamus. Psychiatry Clin Neurosci 1997;51(2):79-81.

Kishi Y, Konishi S, Koizumi S, Kudo Y, Kurosawa H, Kathol RG. Schizophrenia and narcolepsy: a review with a case report. Psychiatry Clin Neurosci 2004;58(2): 117-124.

Krahn LE, Pankratz VS, Oliver L, Boeve BF, Silber MH. Hypocretin (orexin) levels in cerebrospinal fluid of patients with narcolepsy: relationship to cataplexy and HLA DQB1*0602 status. Sleep 2002;25(7):733-736.

Krieger J, Meslier N, Lebrun T, Levy P, Phillip-Joet F, Sailly JC et al. Accidents in obstructive sleep apnea patients treated with nasal continuous positive airway pressure: a prospective study. The Working Group ANTADIR, Paris and CRESGE, Lille, France. Association Nationale de Traitement a Domicile des Insuffisants Respiratoires. Chest 1997;112(6):1561-1566.

Mignot E, Lin X, Arrigoni J, Macaubas C, Olive F, Hallmayer J et al. DQB1*0602 and DQA1*0102 (DQ1) are better markers than DR2 for narcolepsy in Caucasian and black Americans. Sleep 1994;17(8 Suppl):S60-S67.

Mignot E, Nishino S, Guilleminault C, Dement WC. Modafinil binds to the dopamine uptake carrier site with low affinity. Sleep 1994;17(5):436-437.

Mitler MM, Hajdukovic R. Relative efficacy of drugs for the treatment of sleepiness in narcolepsy. Sleep 1991;14(3):218-220.

Morrish E, King MA, Smith IE, Shneerson JM. Factors associated with a delay in the diagnosis of narcolepsy. Sleep Med 2004;5(1):37-41.

Porkka-Heiskanen T, Strecker RE, McCarley RW. Brain site-specificity of extracellular adenosine concentration changes during sleep deprivation and spontaneous sleep: an in vivo microdialysis study. Neuroscience 2000;99(3):507-517.

Qureshi A, Lee-Chiong T, Jr. Medications and their effects on sleep. Med Clin North Am 2004;88(3):751-66, x.

Riley RW, Powell NB, Li KK, Guilleminault CKyger MH, Roth T, Dement WC, editors. Sleep Medicine. 3rd ed Saunders; 2000. p. 913-928.

Sanders MH. Medical Therapy for Obstructive Sleep Apnea-Hypopnea Syndrome. In: Kyger MH, Roth T, Dement WC, editors. Sleep Medicine. 3rd ed Saunders; 2000. p. 879-893.

Sangal RB, Sangal JM. Rating scales for inattention and sleepiness are correlated in adults with symptoms of sleep disordered breathing syndrome, but not in adults with symptoms of attention-deficit/hyperactivity disorder. Sleep Med 2004;5(2):133-135.

Sassani A, Findley LJ, Kryger M, Goldlust E, George C, Davidson TM. Reducing motor-vehicle collisions, costs, and fatalities by treating obstructive sleep apnea syndrome. Sleep 2004;27(3):453-458.

Schneider C, Fulda S, Schulz H. Daytime variation in performance and tiredness/sleepiness ratings in patients with insomnia, narcolepsy, sleep apnea and normal controls. J Sleep Res 2004;13(4):373-383.

Schwartz JR, Nelson MT, Schwartz ER, Hughes RJ. Effects of modafinil on wakefulness and executive function in patients with narcolepsy experiencing late-day sleepiness. Clin Neuropharmacol 2004;27(2):74-79.

Seamans JK, Yang CR. The principal features and mechanisms of dopamine modulation in the prefrontal cortex. Prog Neurobiol 2004;74(1):1-58.

Singewald N, Salchner P, Sharp T. Induction of c-Fos expression in specific areas of the fear circuitry in rat forebrain by anxiogenic drugs. Biol Psychiatry

2003;53(4):275-283.

Sutcliffe JG, de LL. The hypocretins: setting the arousal threshold. Nat Rev Neurosci 2002;3(5):339-349.

Teixeira VG, Faccenda JF, Douglas NJ. Functional status in patients with narcolepsy. Sleep Med 2004;5(5):477-483.

Verstraeten E, Cluydts R. Executive control of attention in sleep apnea patients: theoretical concepts and methodological considerations. Sleep Med Rev 2004;8(4):257-267.

Wesensten NJ, Belenky G, Kautz MA, Thorne DR, Reichardt RM, Balkin TJ. Maintaining alertness and performance during sleep deprivation: modafinil versus caffeine. Psychopharmacology (Berl) 2002;159(3):238-247.

Yang P, Chung LC, Chen CS, Chen CC. Rapid improvement in academic grades following methylphenidate treatment in attention-deficit hyperactivity disorder. Psychiatry Clin Neurosci 2004;58(1):37-41.

Sleep Resources

Academy of Dental Sleep Medicine
1 Westbrook Corporate Center, Suite 920, Westchester, IL 60154
(708) 273-9366 • fax (708) 492-0943
www.dentalsleepmed.org • info@dentalsleepmed.org

American Academy of Neurology
1080 Montreal Ave., St. Paul, MN 55116
 (800) 879-1960 • fax (651) 695-2791
www.aan.com • memberservices@aan.com

American Academy of Sleep Medicine
1 Westbrook Corporate Center, Suite 920, Westchester, IL 60154
(708) 492-0930 • fax (708) 492-0943
www.aasmnet.org

American Board of Sleep Medicine
(708) 492-1290 • fax (708) 492-0942
www.absm.org • absm@absm.org

American Sleep Apnea Association
1424 K Street NW, Suite 302, Washington, DC 20005
(202) 293-3650 • fax (202) 293-3656
www.sleepapnea.org

American Sleep Disorders Association
6301 Bandel Road, Suite 101, Rochester, MN 55901
(507) 287-6006 • fax (507) 287-6008

Associated Professional Sleep Societies, LLC
1 Westbrook Corporate Center, Suite 920, Westchester, IL 60154
(708) 492-0930 • fax (708) 492-0943
www.apss.org

Association of Polysomnographic Technologies
1 Westbrook Corporate Center, Suite 920, Westchester, IL 60154
(708) 492-0796 • fax (708) 273-9344
www.aptweb.org • cwaring@aptweb.org

European Sleep Research Society
Sleep Disorders Unit, Department of Neurology,
Fundación Jiménez Diaz
Avda. de los Reyes Católicos, 2
28040 Madrid, Spain
 +34-91 543 1423 • fax +34-91 543 9316
www.esrs.org • dgarciaborreguero@fjd.es

International Sleep Products Association
501 Wythe Street, Alexandria, VA 22314
(703) 683-8371 • fax (703) 683-4503
www.sleepproducts.org • info@sleepproducts.org

Narcolepsy Network, Inc.
PO Box 294, Pleasantville, NY 10570
(401) 667-2523 • fax (401) 633-6567
www.narcolepsynetwork.org • narnet@narcolepsynetwork.org

National Foundation for Sleep and Related Disorders in Children
4200 W. Peterson, Suite 109, Chicago, IL 60646
(708) 971-1086 • fax (312) 434-5311

National Sleep Foundation
1552 K Street, NW, Suite 500, Washington, DC 20005
(202) 347-3471 • fax (202) 347-3472
www.sleepfoundation.org • NSF@sleepfoundation.org

Sleep Medicine Research Foundation
4475 Paradenton Avenue, Dublin, OH 43017
(614) 766-0773 • fax (614) 766-2599

Sleep Research Society
1 Westbrook Corporate Center, Suite 920, Westchester, IL 60154
(708) 492-1093
www.sleepresearchsociety.org • kmcnamara@srsnet.org

Society for Light Treatment and Biological Rhythms
PO Box 591687, 174 Cook Street, San Francisco, CA 94159
Fax (415) 751-2758
www.websciences.org/sltbr • stlbrinfo@al.com

Society for Neuroscience
11 Dupont Circle, NW, Suite 500, Washington, DC 20036
(202) 462-6688 • fax (202) 462-9740
http://apu.sfn.org • info@sfn.org

Society for Research on Biological Rhythms
University of Illinois at Urbana-Champaign
162 Administration Building, 506 S. Wright Street, Urbana, IL 61801
(217) 333-2880 • fax (217) 333-9561
www.srbr.org • klp68@ad.uiuc.edu

Index

About the Author

Stephen M. Stahl, M.D., Ph.D.

Chairman, Neuroscience Education Institute
and Adjunct Professor, University of California, San Diego

Dr. Stephen M. Stahl received his undergraduate and medical degrees from Northwestern University in Chicago, as a member of the honors program in Medical Education, and his Ph.D. degree in pharmacology and physiology from the University of Chicago. Dr. Stahl is trained in three specialties: internal medicine at the University of Chicago; neurology at the University of California in San Francisco; and psychiatry at Stanford University. He is board certified in psychiatry.

Dr. Stahl has held faculty positions at Stanford University, the University of California at Los Angeles, the Institute of Psychiatry London, the Institute of Neurology London, and, currently, as Adjunct Professor of Psychiatry at the University of California at San Diego. Dr. Stahl was also Executive Director of Clinical Neurosciences at the Merck Neuroscience Research Center in the UK for several years. Now Dr. Stahl serves as Chairman of the Neuroscience Education Institute (NEI), a medical education center dedicated to producing and disseminating information about diseases and their treatments in psychiatry and neurology, with a special emphasis on multimedia, the internet, and teaching how to teach.

During his career, Dr. Stahl has conducted numerous research projects, awarded by the National Institute of Mental Health, by the Veterans Administration, and by the pharmaceutical industry. Author of more than 350 articles and chapters, Dr. Stahl is an internationally recognized clinician, researcher, and teacher in psychiatry with subspecialty expertise in psychopharmacology. Dr. Stahl has edited two books, and written four others, including the best-selling textbook, *Essential Psychopharmacology*, now in its second edition, and the recently published *Essential Psychopharmacology: The Prescriber's Guide*.

Lectures, courses, and preceptorships based upon his textbook have taken him to dozens of countries on six continents to speak to tens of thousands of physicians, mental health professionals, and students at all levels. His lectures and scientific presentations have been distributed through more than a million CD-ROMs, internet educational programs, videotapes, audiotapes, and programmed home study texts for continuing medical education to hundreds of thousands of professionals in many different languages. His courses and award-winning multimedia teaching materials are used by psychopharmacology teachers and students throughout the world. Dr. Stahl also writes didactic features for mental health professionals and serves as Editor in Chief of NEI's newsletter, *Psychopharmacology Educational Update*

(*PsychEd Up*). He has been named recipient of the 2002 International College of Neuropsychopharmacology (CINP) Lundbeck Foundation Award in Education for his contributions to postgraduate education in psychiatry and neurology, and is also the winner of the A.E. Bennett Award of the Society of Biological Psychiatry, the 2004 American Psychiatric Association/San Diego Psychiatric Society Education Award, and has been cited as both one of "America's Top Psychiatrists" and one of the "Best Doctors in America."

Dr. Stahl serves as a fellow of the ACNP (American College of Neuropsychopharmacology) and as vice president of the CINP. He serves on numerous editorial boards including clinical field editor for the *International Journal of Neuropsychopharmacology*. He also serves on numerous medical and scientific advisory boards for the pharmaceutical industry, for the biotechnology and medical information industry, and for various nonprofit and public service organizations, including appointment by the State of California to the Medi-Cal Oversight Board for Medicines (Drug Utilization Review Board).

His current research program includes studies on how to identify and reduce variance in psychopharmacology ratings for multi-center trials through the use of multimedia and internet-based rater training programs. He is also investigating the use of antipsychotic drugs in the public health sector of California, utilizing physician education rather than formulary restrictions to reduce high cost low evidence based uses of these agents. Other educational research programs are monitoring changes in diagnosing and prescribing behaviors as outcomes from various educational interventions for NEI programs. He is an active clinical investigator for a wide variety of psychopharmacologic agents and has a clinical practice specializing in psychopharmacologic treatment of resistant cases.